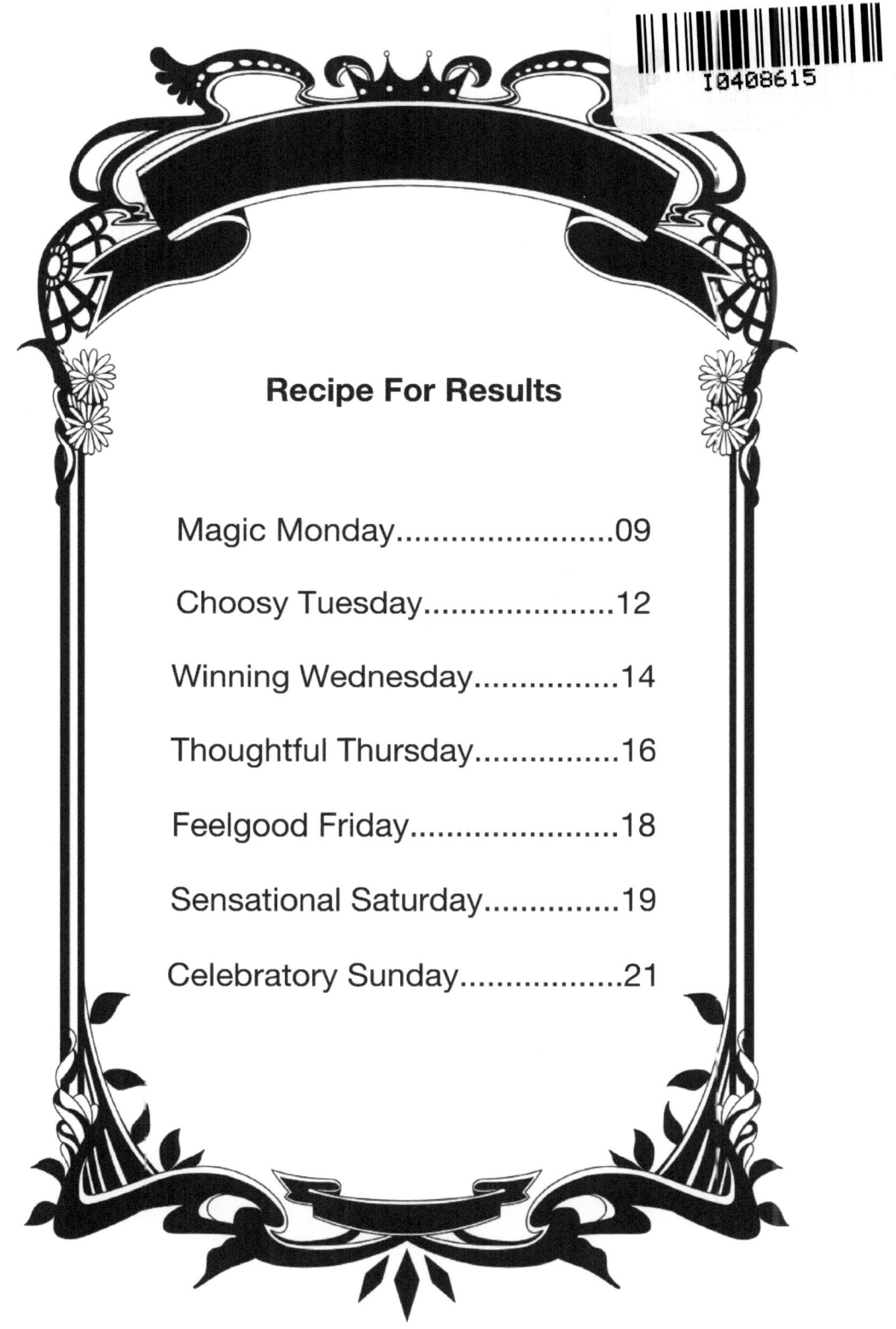

## Recipe For Results

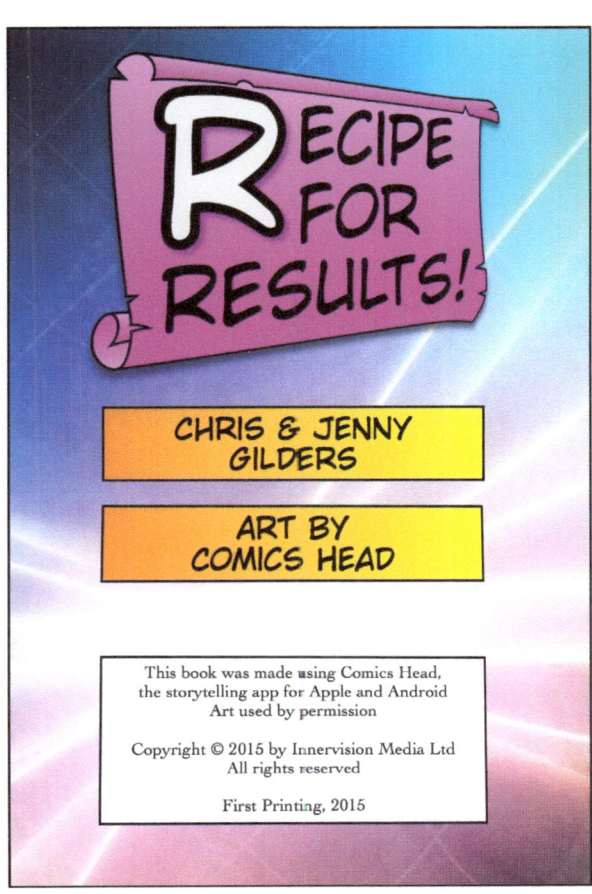

# RECIPE FOR RESULTS!

**CHRIS & JENNY GILDERS**

**ART BY COMICS HEAD**

This book was made using Comics Head, the storytelling app for Apple and Android Art used by permission

First Printing, 2015

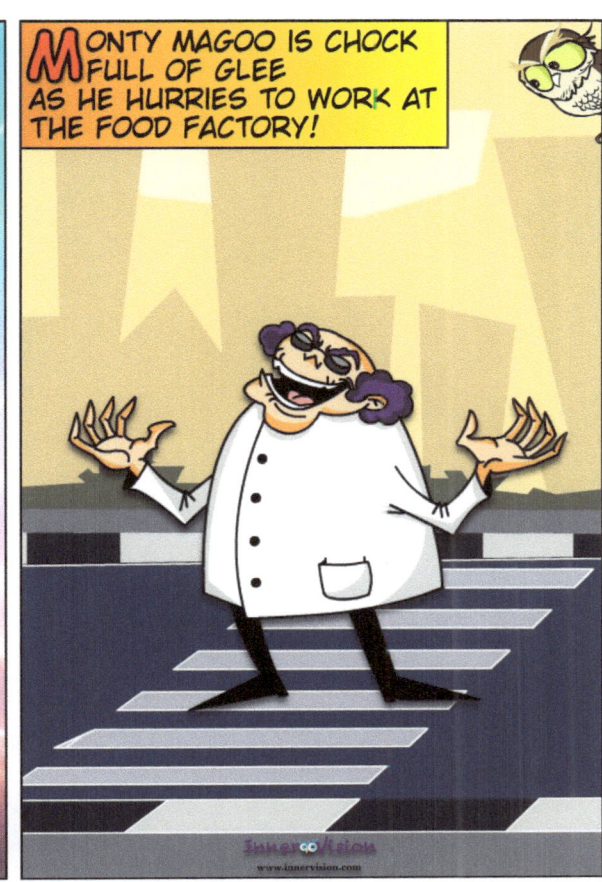

MONTY MAGOO IS CHOCK FULL OF GLEE AS HE HURRIES TO WORK AT THE FOOD FACTORY!

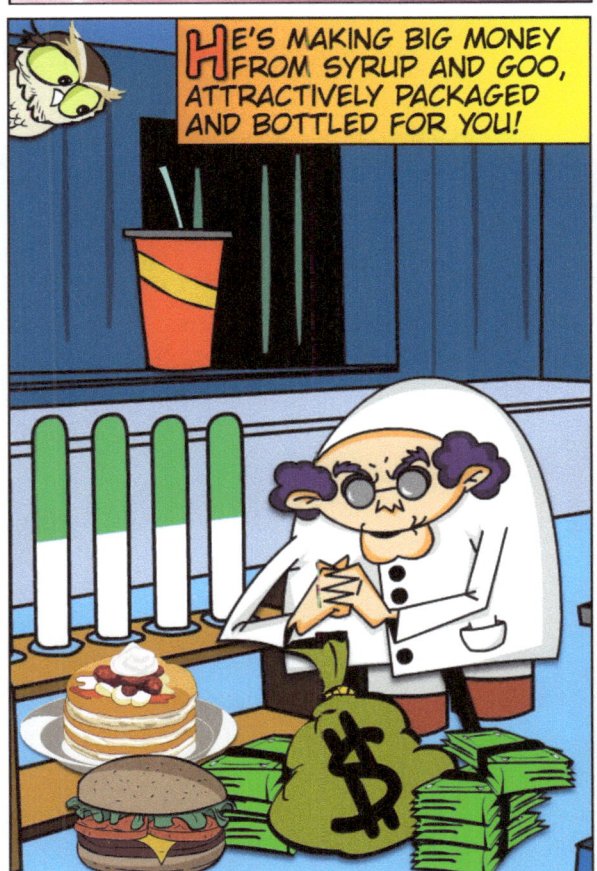

HE'S MAKING BIG MONEY FROM SYRUP AND GOO, ATTRACTIVELY PACKAGED AND BOTTLED FOR YOU!

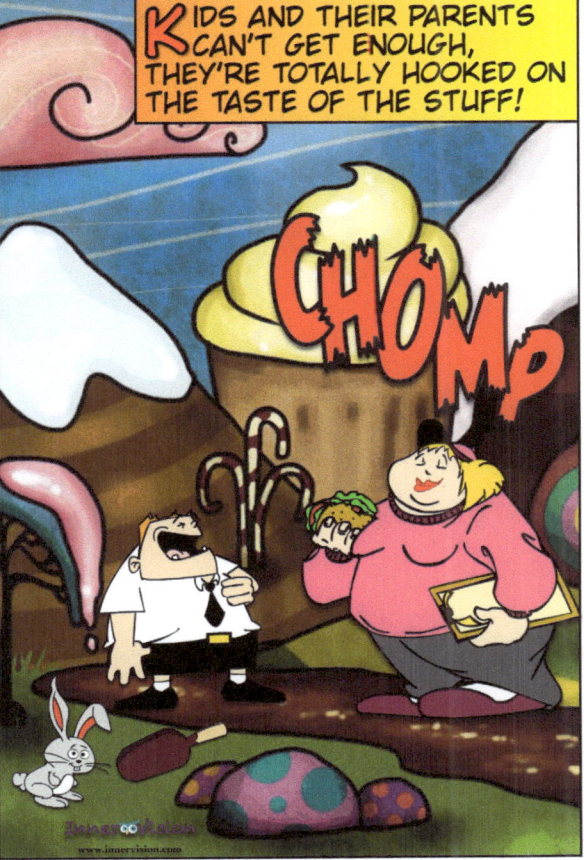

KIDS AND THEIR PARENTS CAN'T GET ENOUGH, THEY'RE TOTALLY HOOKED ON THE TASTE OF THE STUFF!

CHOMP

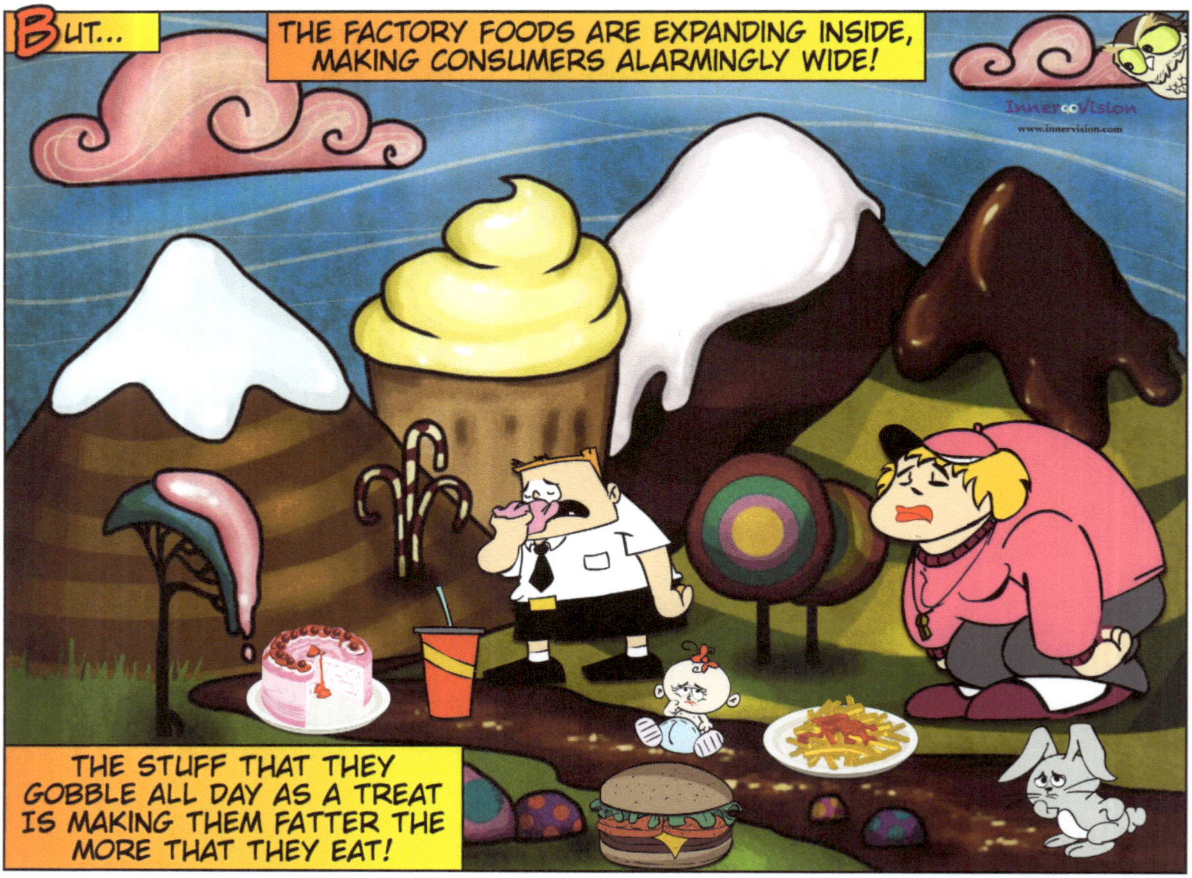

**B**UT... THE FACTORY FOODS ARE EXPANDING INSIDE, MAKING CONSUMERS ALARMINGLY WIDE!

THE STUFF THAT THEY GOBBLE ALL DAY AS A TREAT IS MAKING THEM FATTER THE MORE THAT THEY EAT!

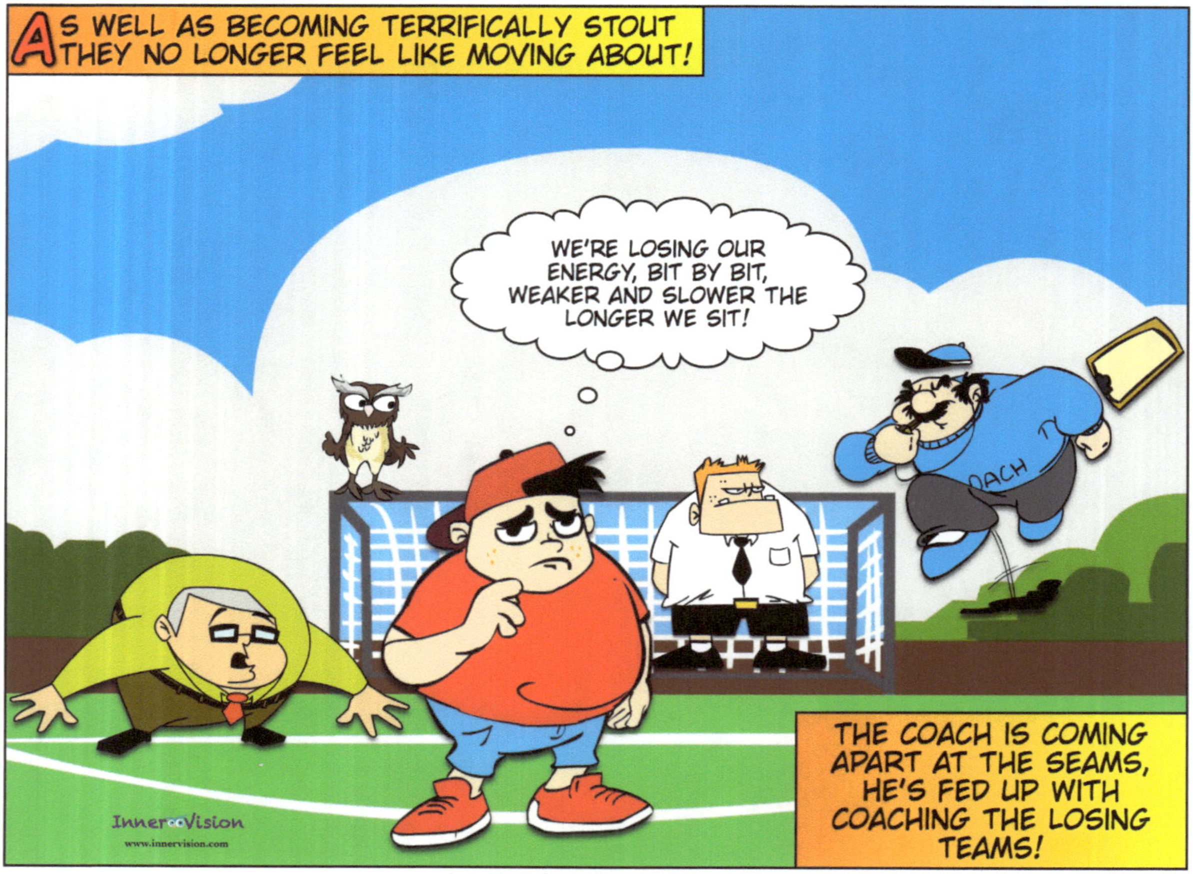

**A**S WELL AS BECOMING TERRIFICALLY STOUT THEY NO LONGER FEEL LIKE MOVING ABOUT!

WE'RE LOSING OUR ENERGY, BIT BY BIT, WEAKER AND SLOWER THE LONGER WE SIT!

THE COACH IS COMING APART AT THE SEAMS, HE'S FED UP WITH COACHING THE LOSING TEAMS!

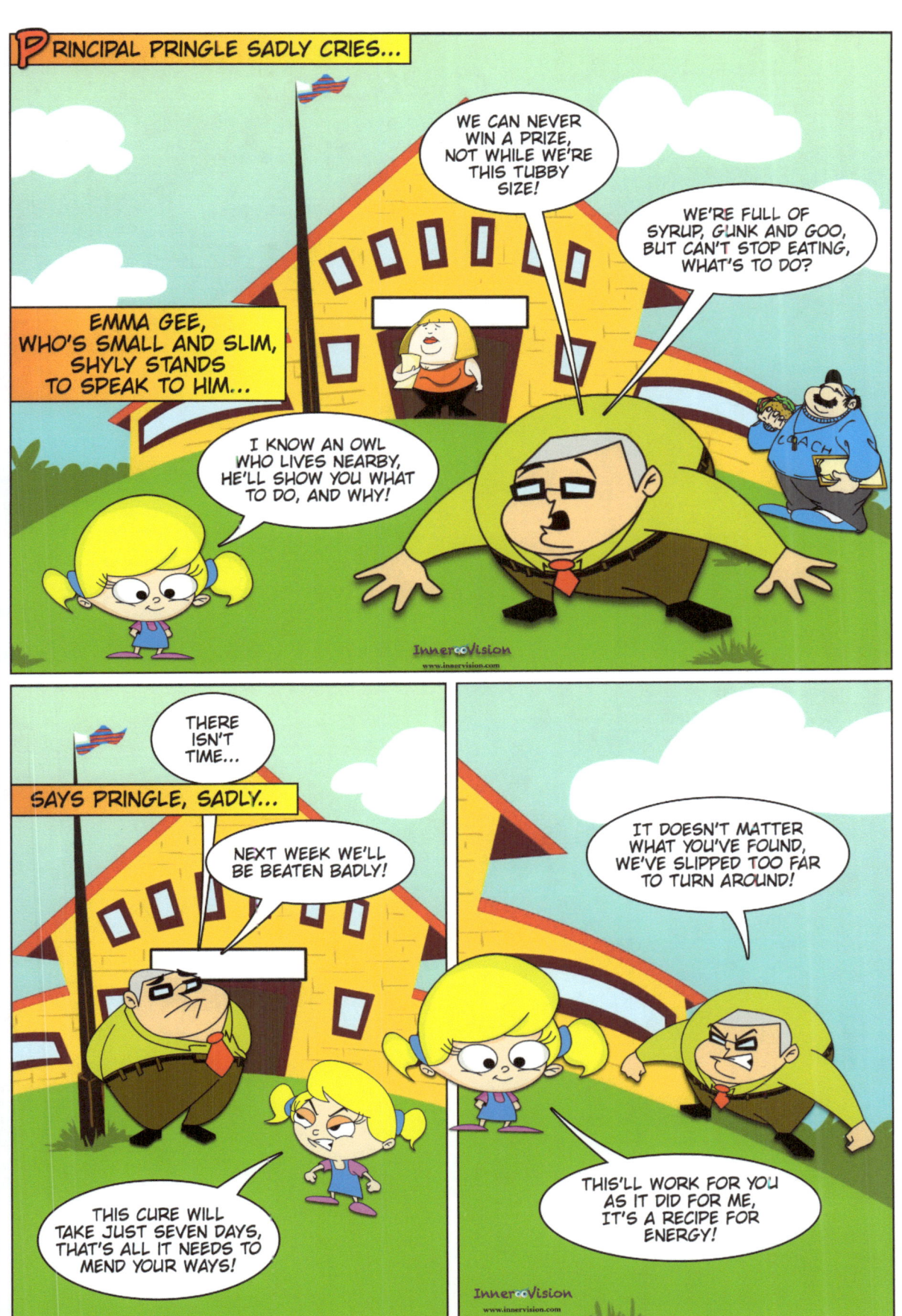

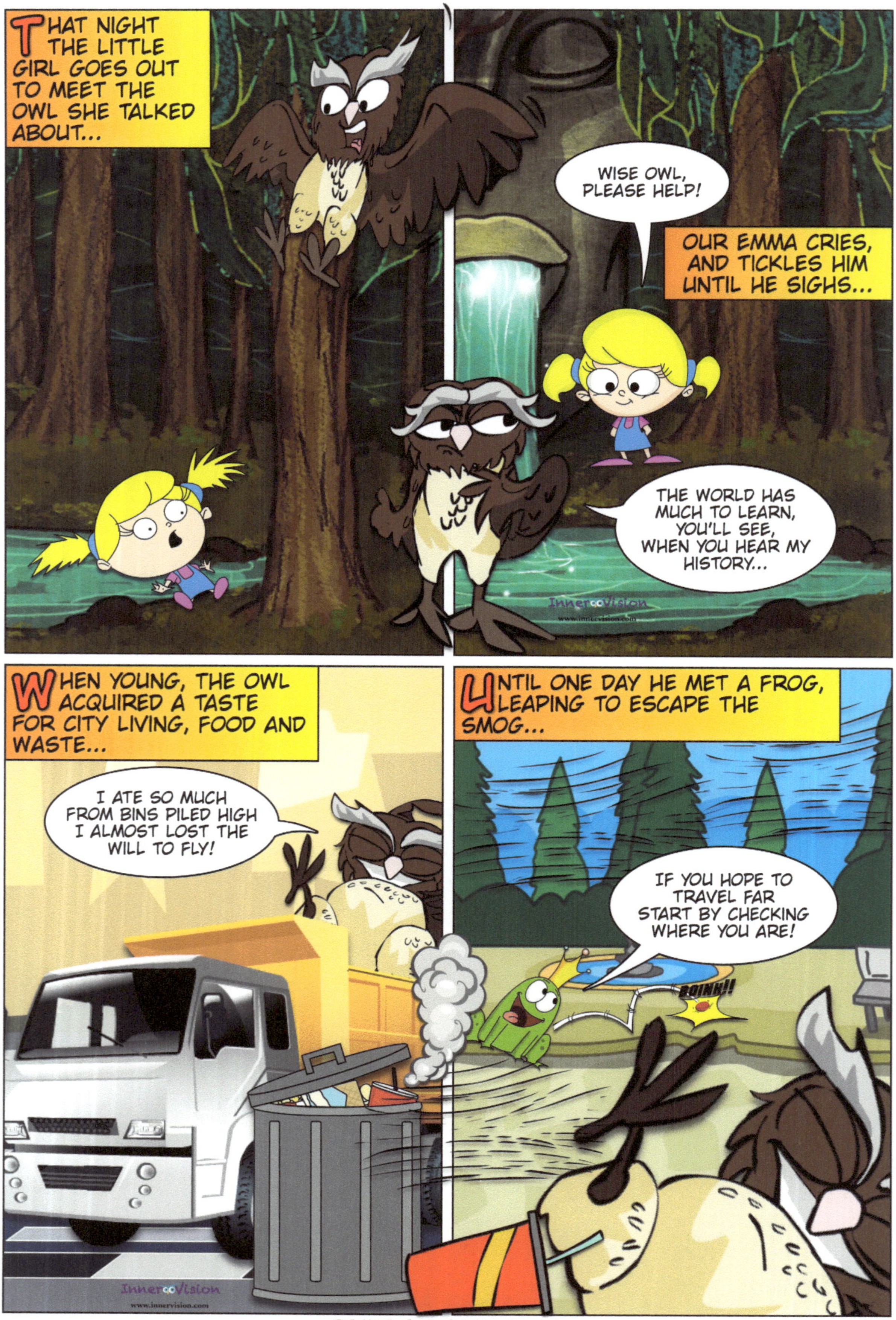

THAT NIGHT THE LITTLE GIRL GOES OUT TO MEET THE OWL SHE TALKED ABOUT...

WISE OWL, PLEASE HELP!

OUR EMMA CRIES, AND TICKLES HIM UNTIL HE SIGHS...

THE WORLD HAS MUCH TO LEARN, YOU'LL SEE, WHEN YOU HEAR MY HISTORY...

WHEN YOUNG, THE OWL ACQUIRED A TASTE FOR CITY LIVING, FOOD AND WASTE...

I ATE SO MUCH FROM BINS PILED HIGH I ALMOST LOST THE WILL TO FLY!

UNTIL ONE DAY HE MET A FROG, LEAPING TO ESCAPE THE SMOG...

IF YOU HOPE TO TRAVEL FAR START BY CHECKING WHERE YOU ARE!

BOINK!!

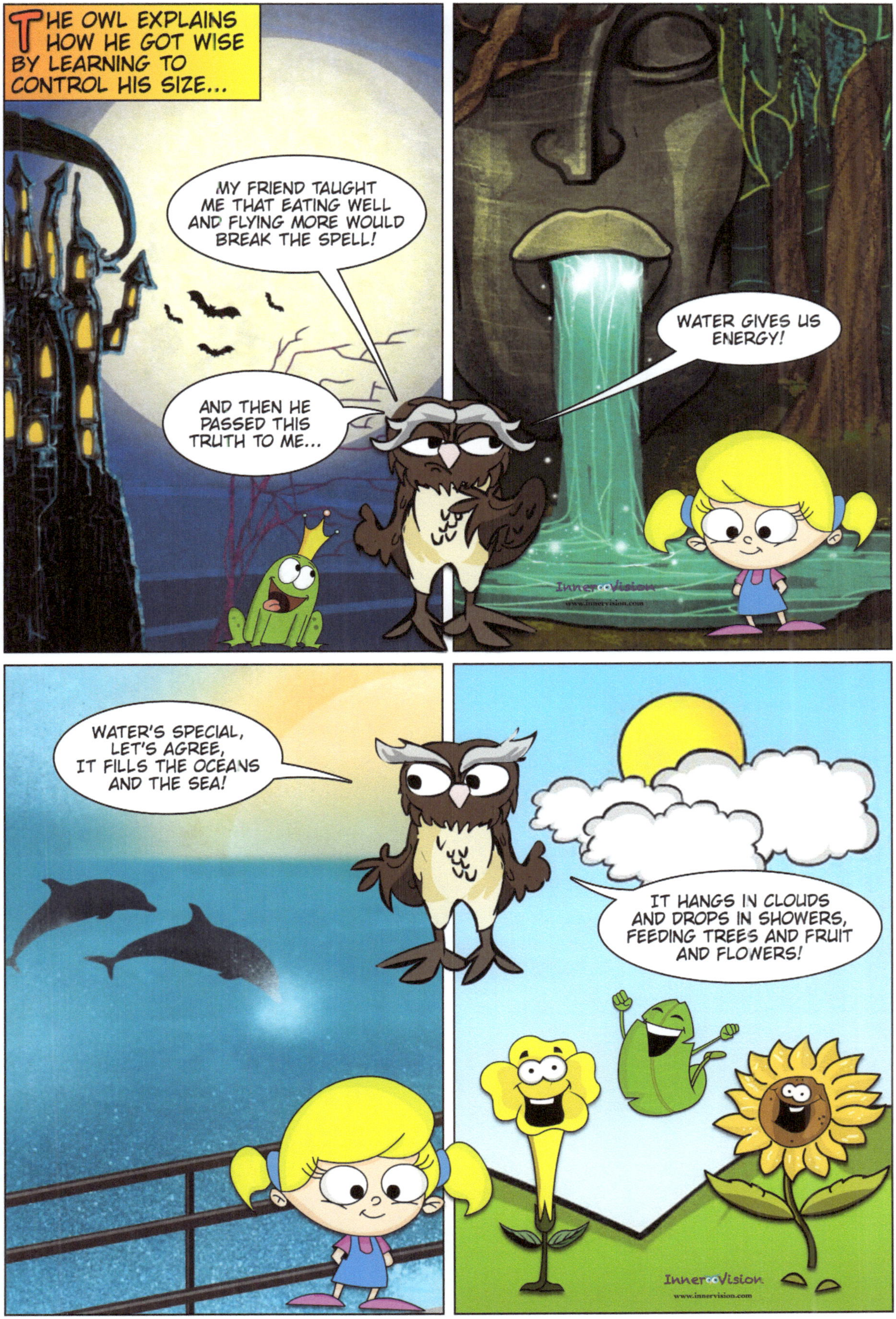
THE OWL EXPLAINS HOW HE GOT WISE BY LEARNING TO CONTROL HIS SIZE...
MY FRIEND TAUGHT ME THAT EATING WELL AND FLYING MORE WOULD BREAK THE SPELL!
AND THEN HE PASSED THIS TRUTH TO ME...
WATER GIVES US ENERGY!
InnerVision
www.innervision.com
WATER'S SPECIAL, LET'S AGREE, IT FILLS THE OCEANS AND THE SEA!
IT HANGS IN CLOUDS AND DROPS IN SHOWERS, FEEDING TREES AND FRUIT AND FLOWERS!
InnerVision
www.innervision.com

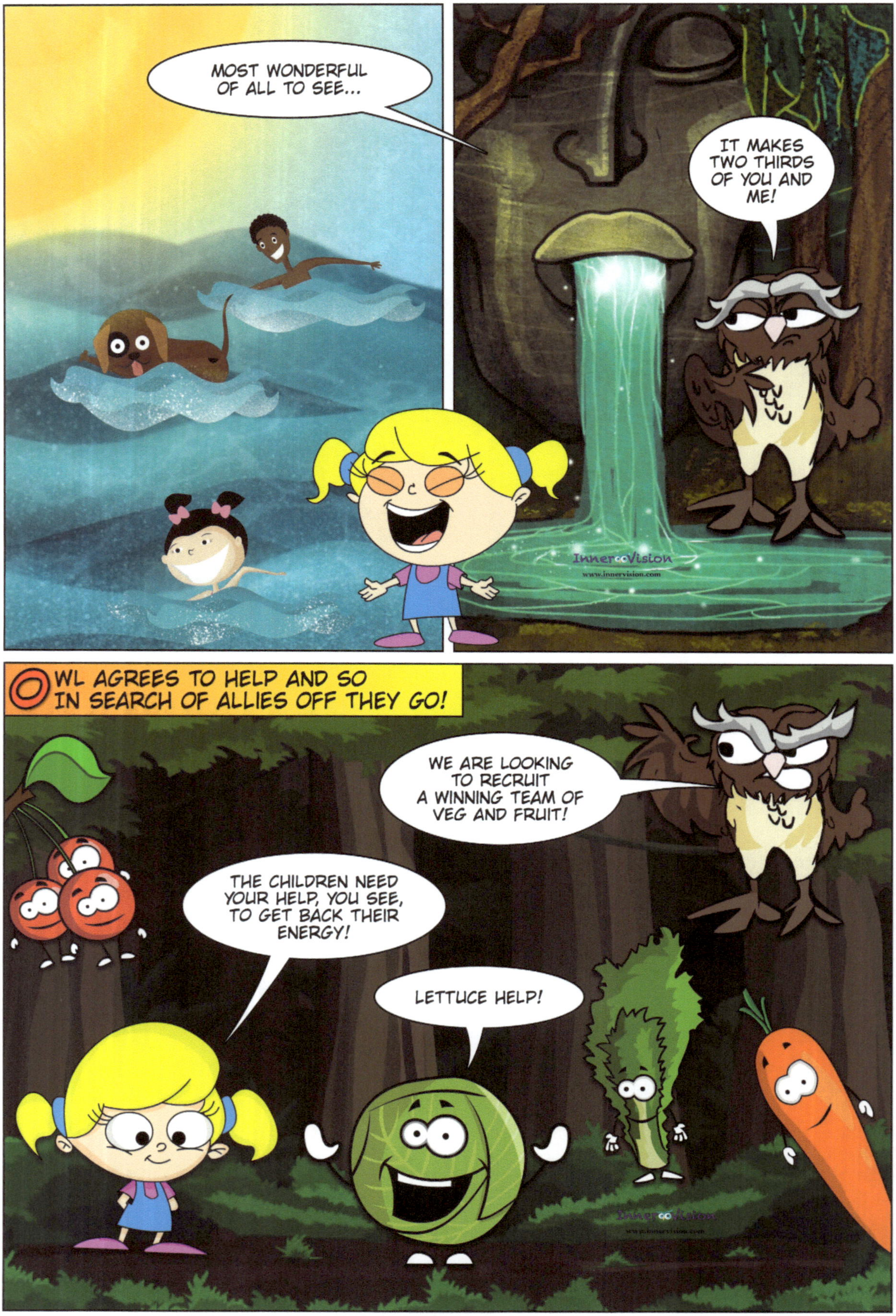

MOST WONDERFUL OF ALL TO SEE...

IT MAKES TWO THIRDS OF YOU AND ME!

OWL AGREES TO HELP AND SO IN SEARCH OF ALLIES OFF THEY GO!

WE ARE LOOKING TO RECRUIT A WINNING TEAM OF VEG AND FRUIT!

THE CHILDREN NEED YOUR HELP, YOU SEE, TO GET BACK THEIR ENERGY!

LETTUCE HELP!

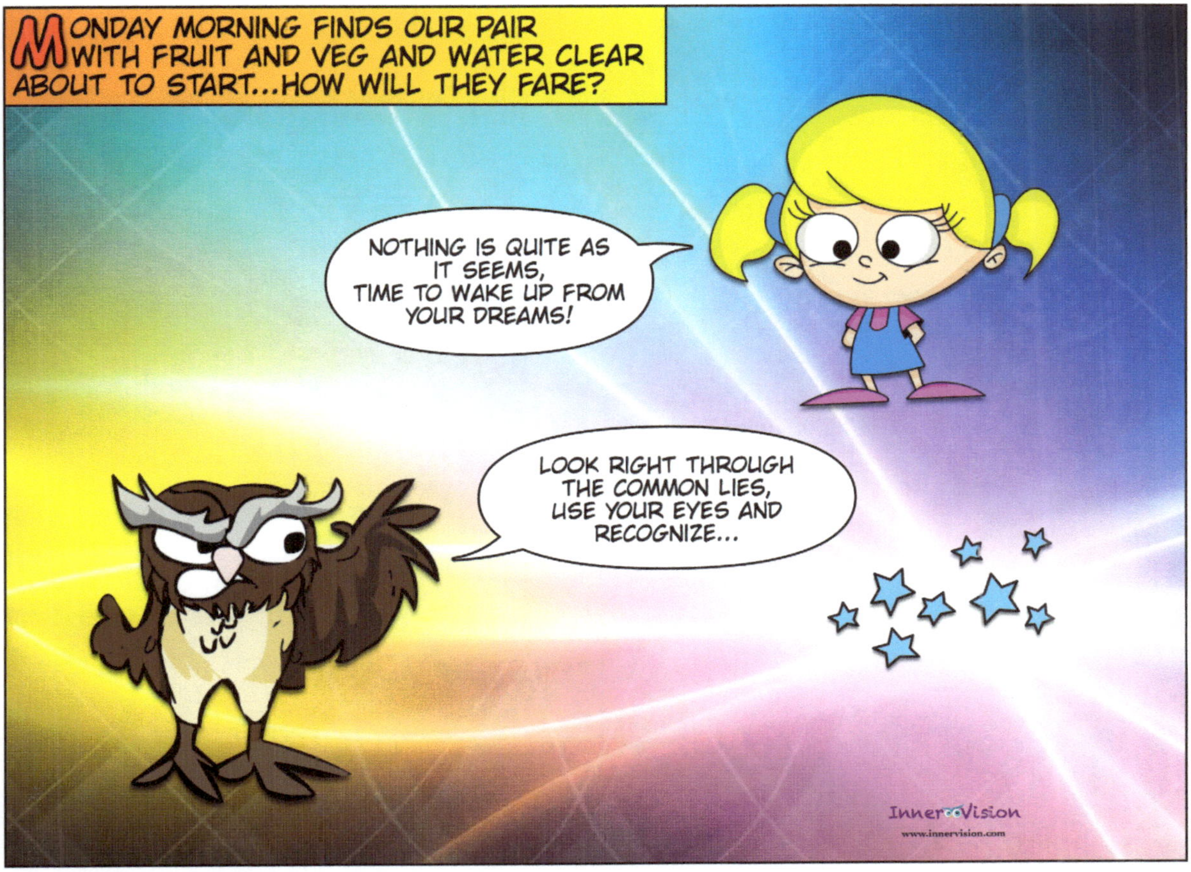

MONDAY MORNING FINDS OUR PAIR WITH FRUIT AND VEG AND WATER CLEAR ABOUT TO START...HOW WILL THEY FARE?

NOTHING IS QUITE AS IT SEEMS, TIME TO WAKE UP FROM YOUR DREAMS!

LOOK RIGHT THROUGH THE COMMON LIES, USE YOUR EYES AND RECOGNIZE...

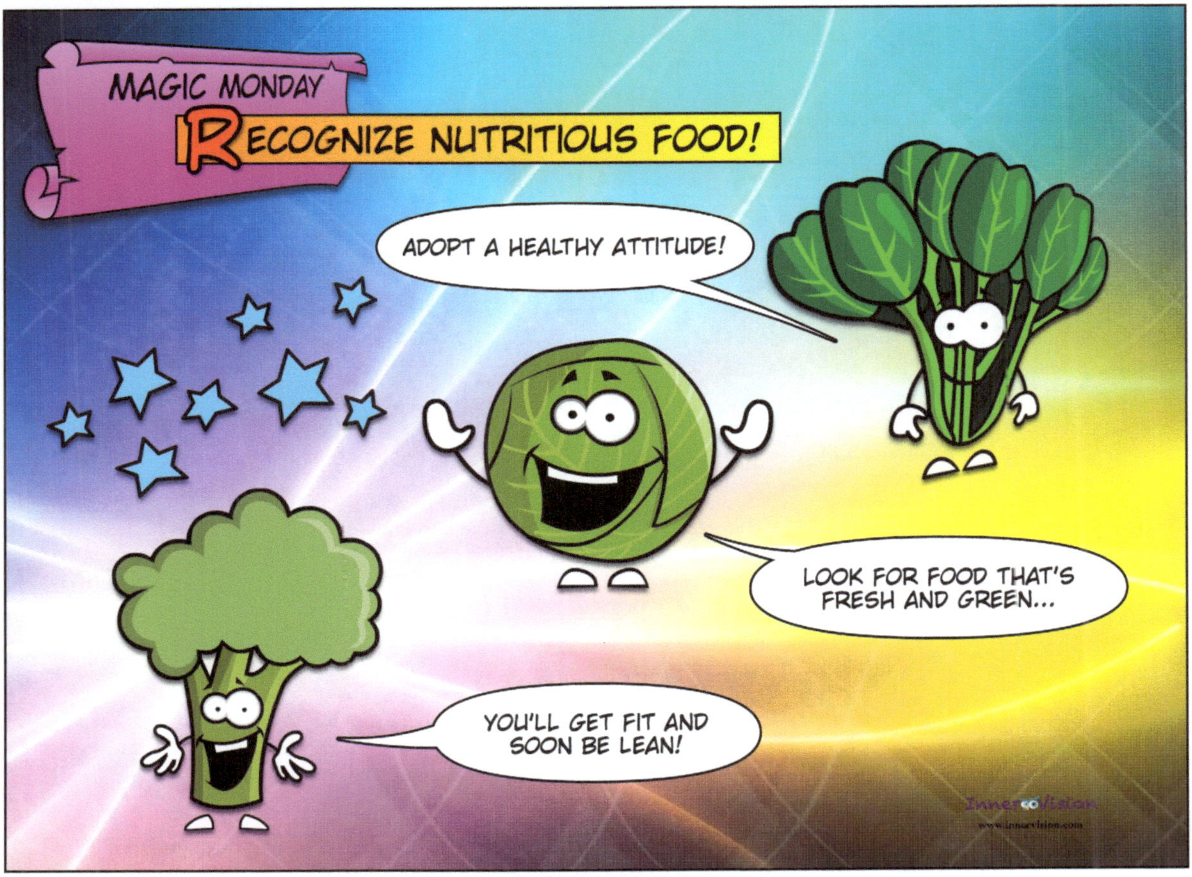

MAGIC MONDAY
RECOGNIZE NUTRITIOUS FOOD!

ADOPT A HEALTHY ATTITUDE!

LOOK FOR FOOD THAT'S FRESH AND GREEN...

YOU'LL GET FIT AND SOON BE LEAN!

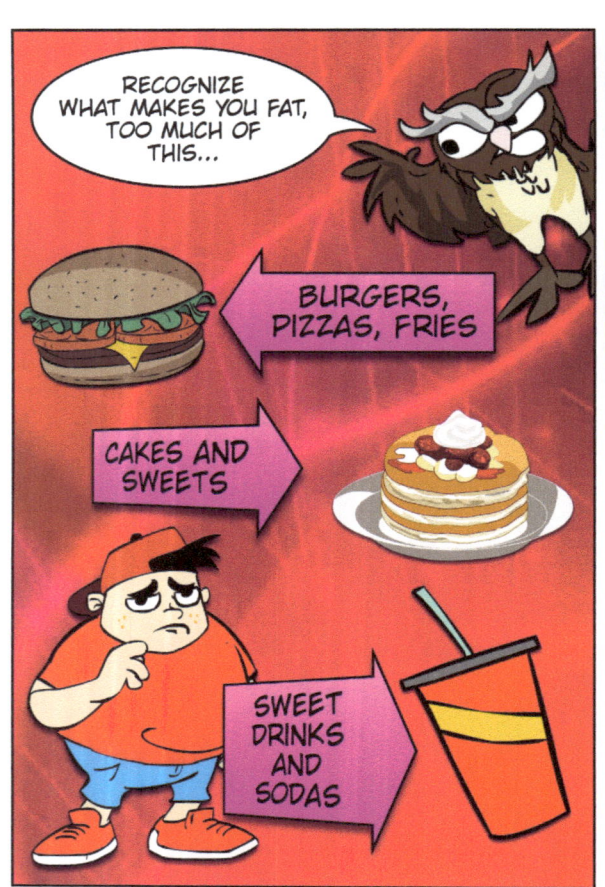

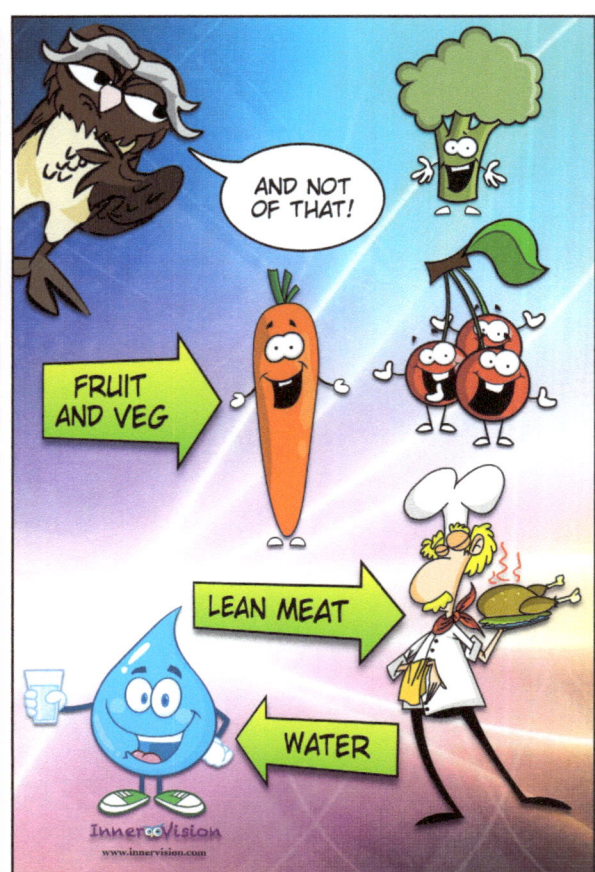

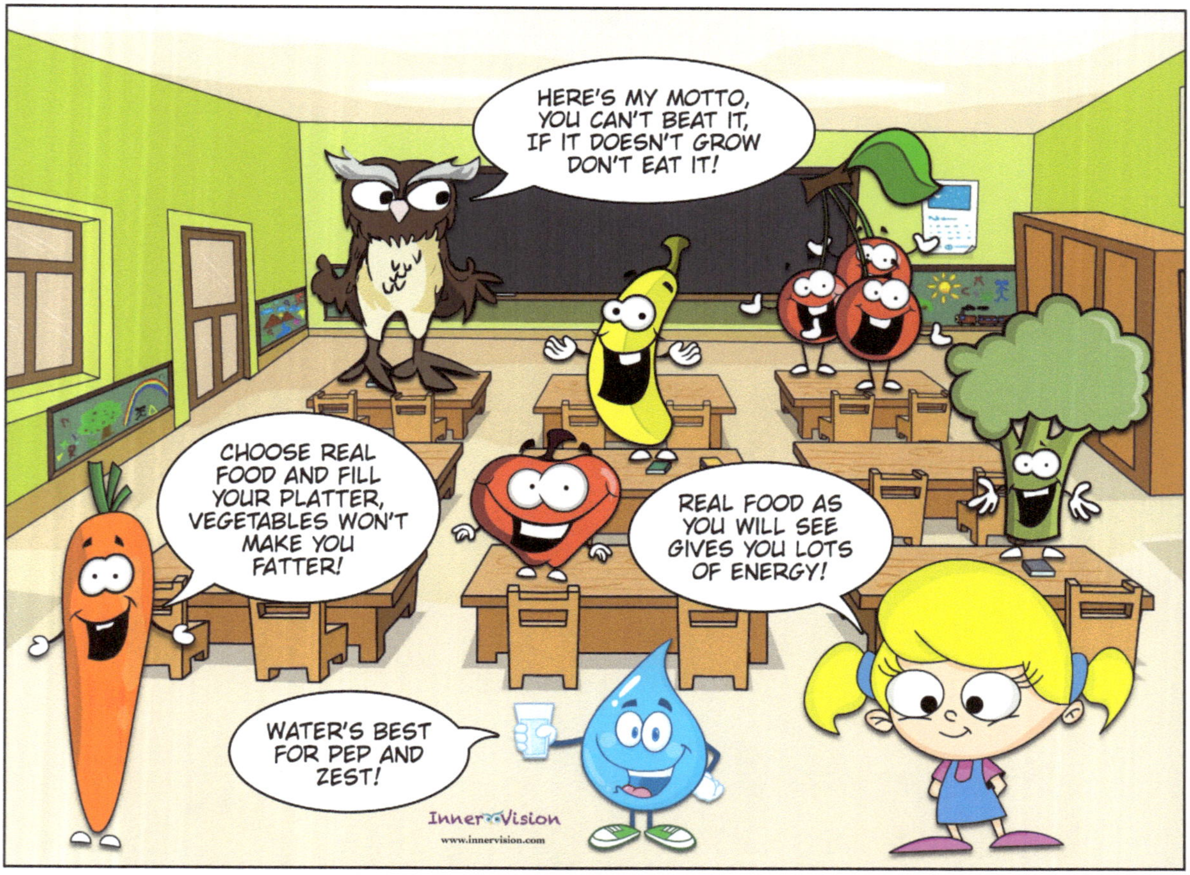

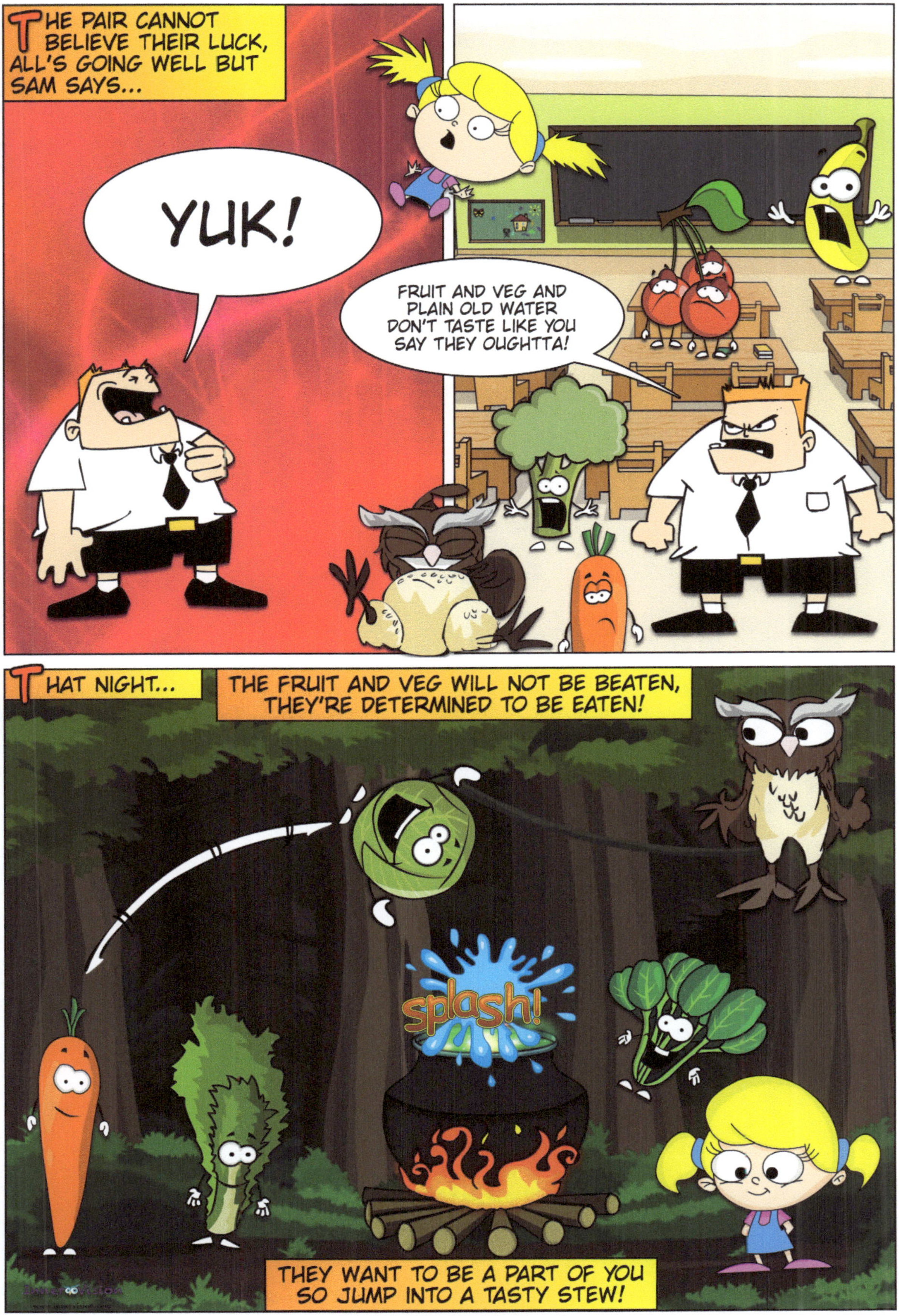

THE PAIR CANNOT BELIEVE THEIR LUCK, ALL'S GOING WELL BUT SAM SAYS...

YUK!

FRUIT AND VEG AND PLAIN OLD WATER DON'T TASTE LIKE YOU SAY THEY OUGHTTA!

THAT NIGHT... THE FRUIT AND VEG WILL NOT BE BEATEN, THEY'RE DETERMINED TO BE EATEN!

splash!

THEY WANT TO BE A PART OF YOU SO JUMP INTO A TASTY STEW!

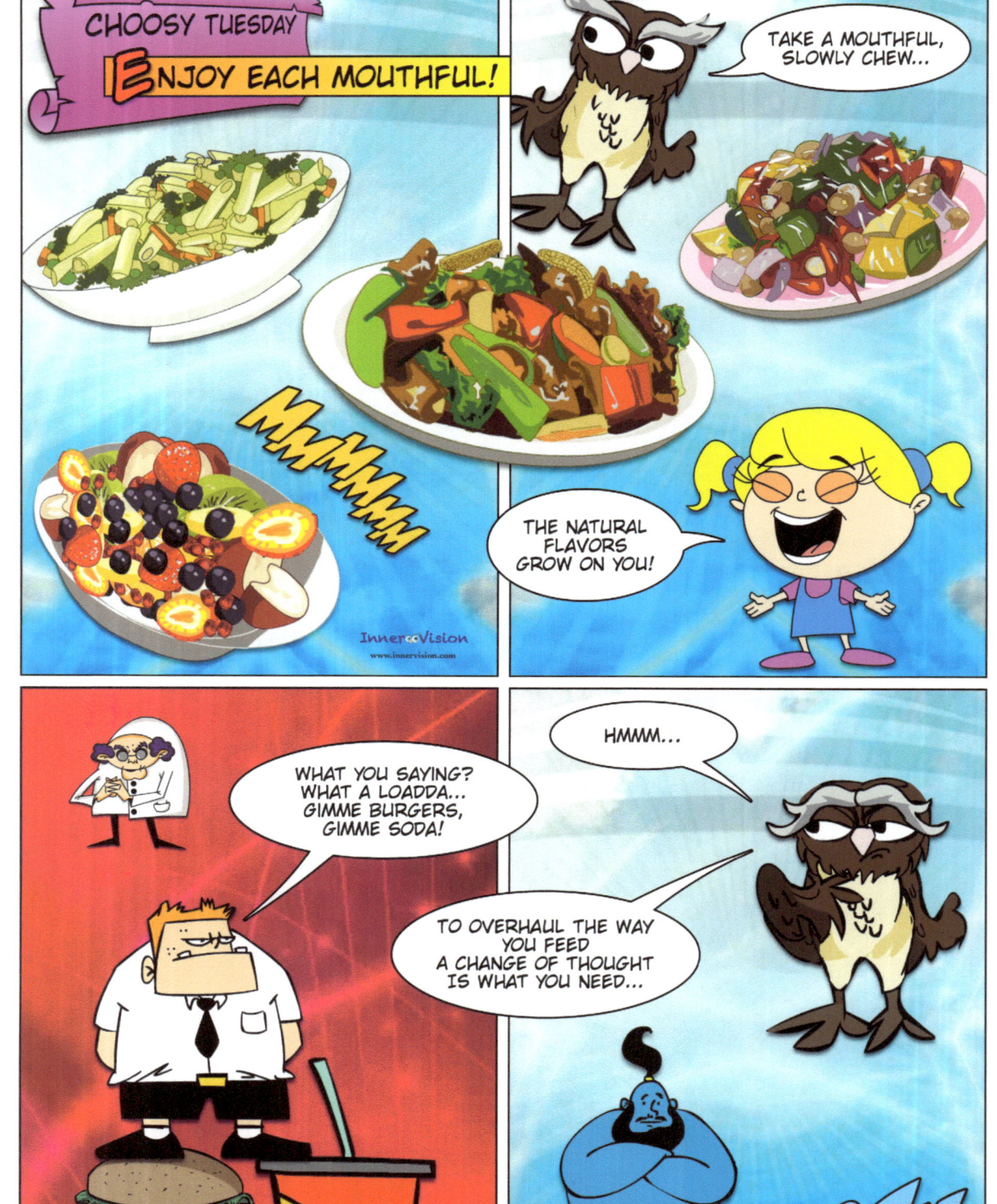

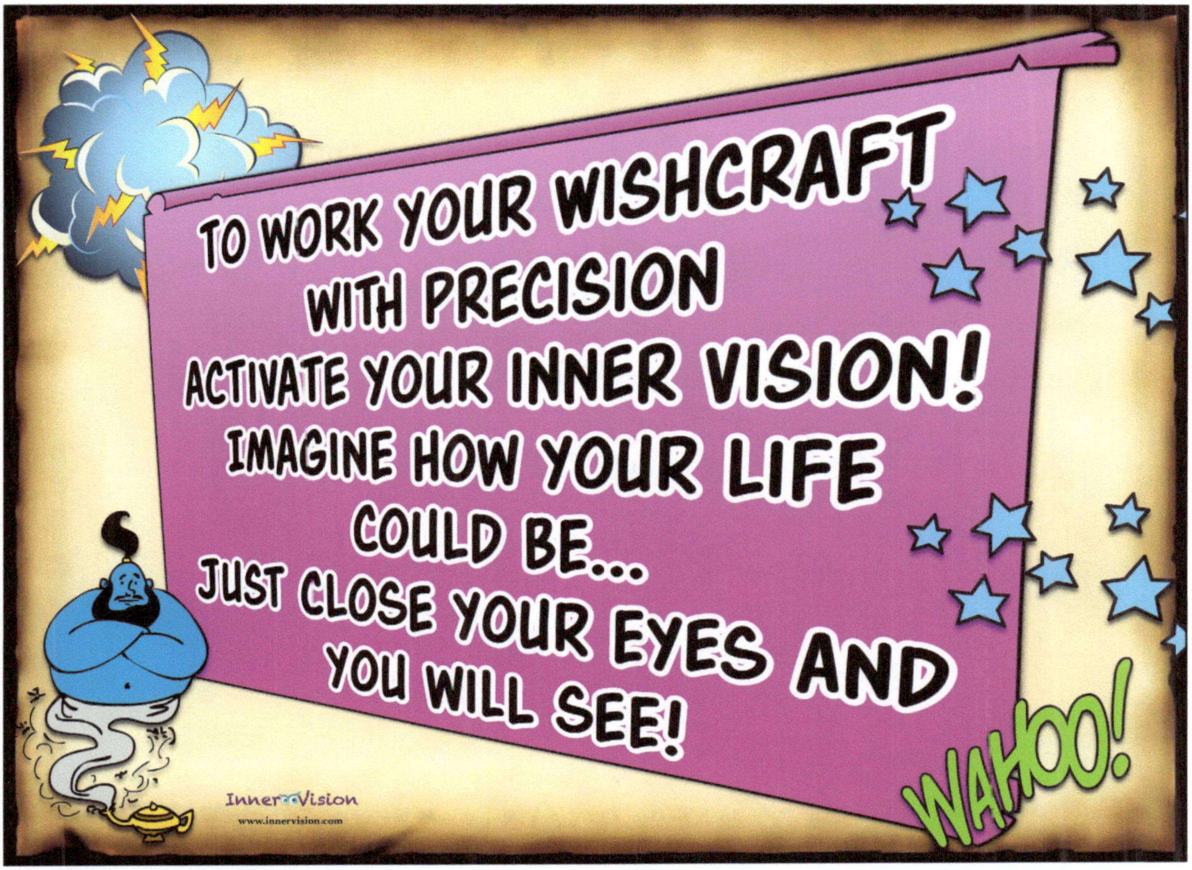
TO WORK YOUR WISHCRAFT
WITH PRECISION
ACTIVATE YOUR INNER VISION!
IMAGINE HOW YOUR LIFE
COULD BE...
JUST CLOSE YOUR EYES AND
YOU WILL SEE!
WAHOO!
InnerVision
www.innervision.com

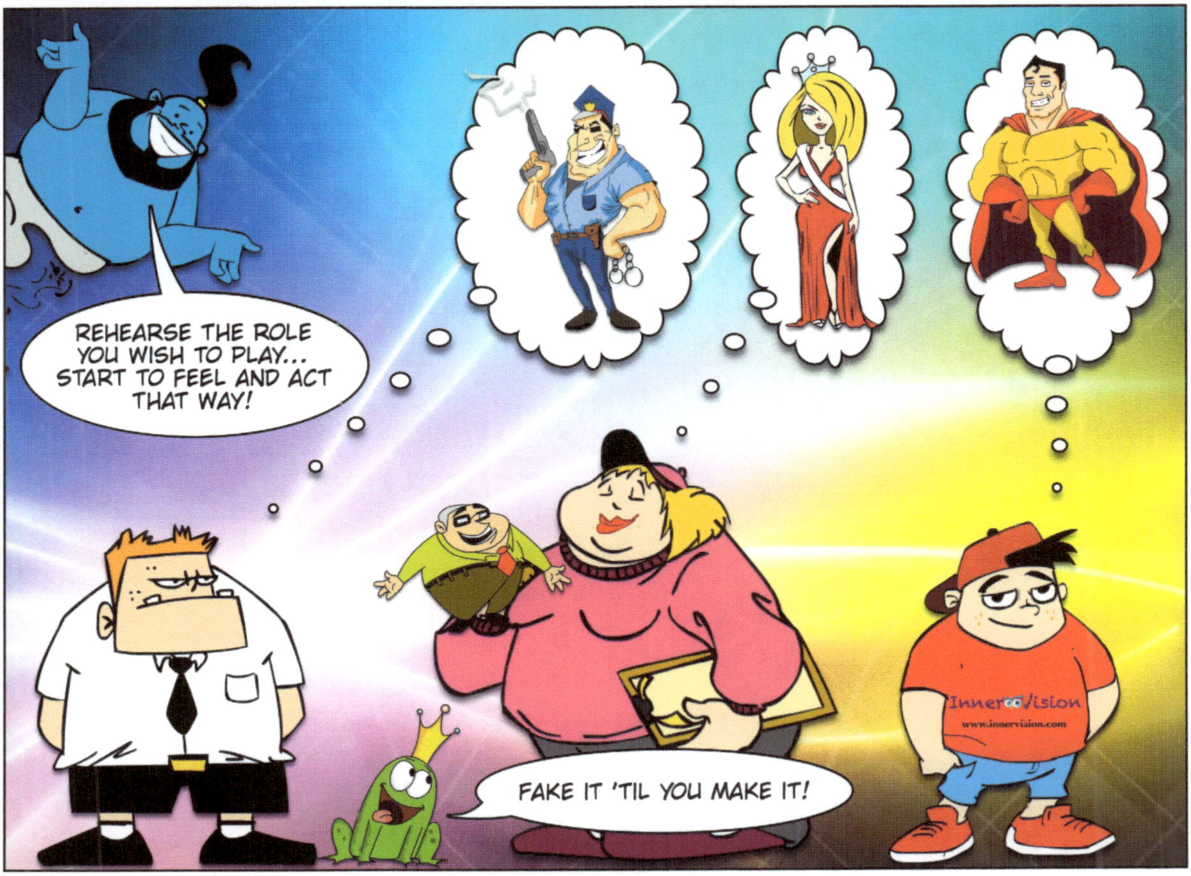
REHEARSE THE ROLE
YOU WISH TO PLAY...
START TO FEEL AND ACT
THAT WAY!
InnerVision
www.innervision.com
FAKE IT 'TIL YOU MAKE IT!

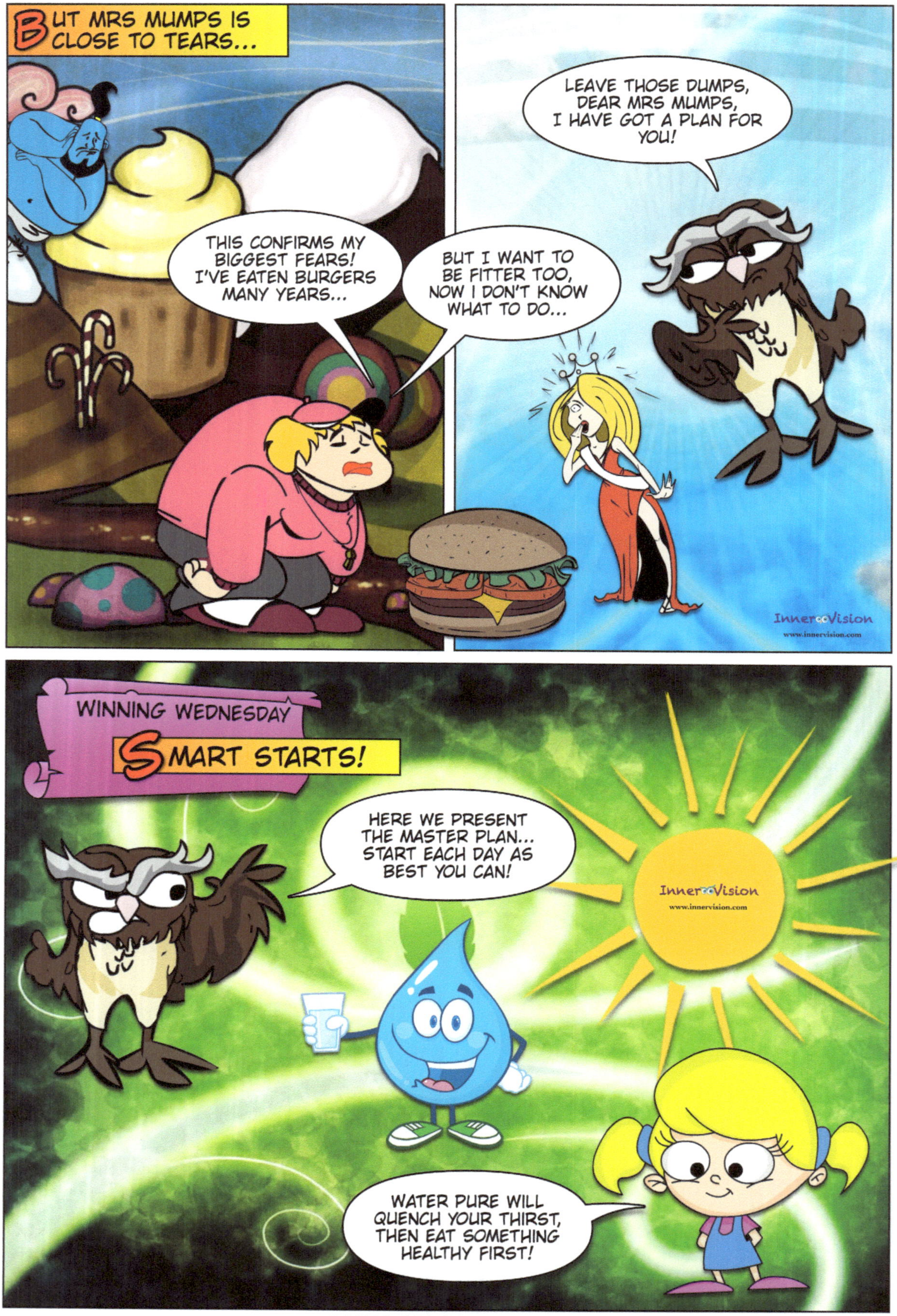
BUT MRS MUMPS IS CLOSE TO TEARS...
THIS CONFIRMS MY BIGGEST FEARS! I'VE EATEN BURGERS MANY YEARS...
BUT I WANT TO BE FITTER TOO, NOW I DON'T KNOW WHAT TO DO...
LEAVE THOSE DUMPS, DEAR MRS MUMPS, I HAVE GOT A PLAN FOR YOU!
InnerVision
www.innervision.com
WINNING WEDNESDAY
SMART STARTS!
HERE WE PRESENT THE MASTER PLAN... START EACH DAY AS BEST YOU CAN!
InnerVision
www.innervision.com
WATER PURE WILL QUENCH YOUR THIRST, THEN EAT SOMETHING HEALTHY FIRST!

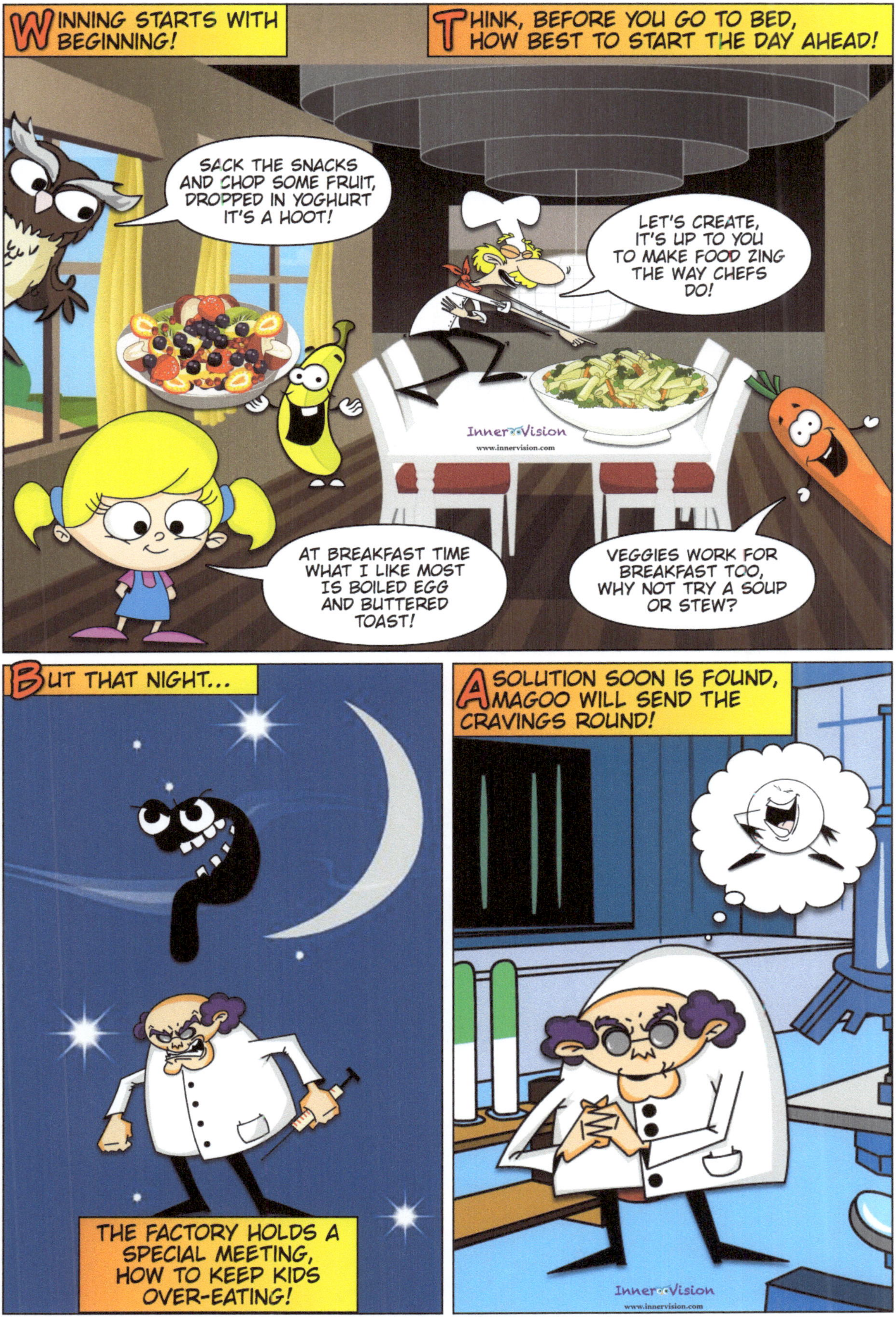

**W**INNING STARTS WITH BEGINNING!

**T**HINK, BEFORE YOU GO TO BED, HOW BEST TO START THE DAY AHEAD!

SACK THE SNACKS AND CHOP SOME FRUIT, DROPPED IN YOGHURT IT'S A HOOT!

LET'S CREATE, IT'S UP TO YOU TO MAKE FOOD ZING THE WAY CHEFS DO!

AT BREAKFAST TIME WHAT I LIKE MOST IS BOILED EGG AND BUTTERED TOAST!

VEGGIES WORK FOR BREAKFAST TOO, WHY NOT TRY A SOUP OR STEW?

Inner Vision
www.innervision.com

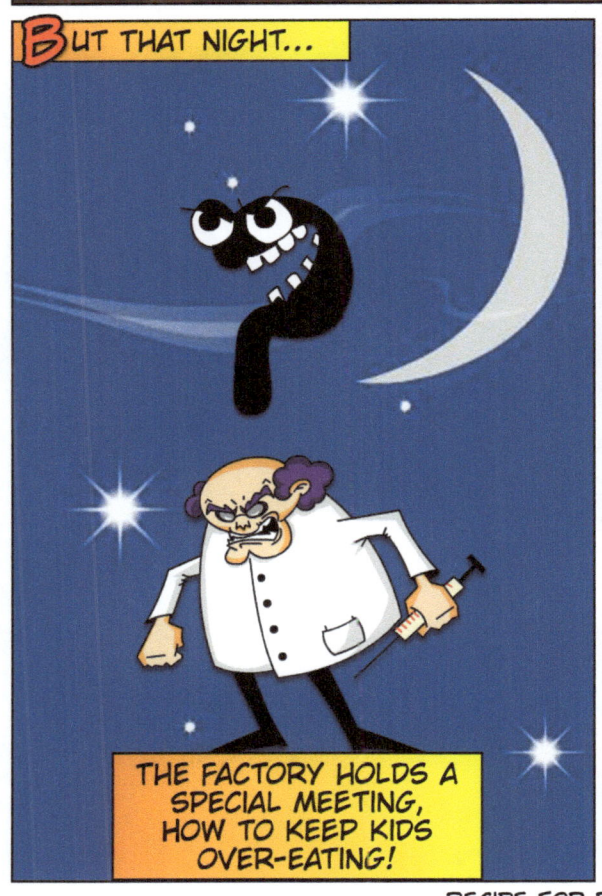

**B**UT THAT NIGHT...

THE FACTORY HOLDS A SPECIAL MEETING, HOW TO KEEP KIDS OVER-EATING!

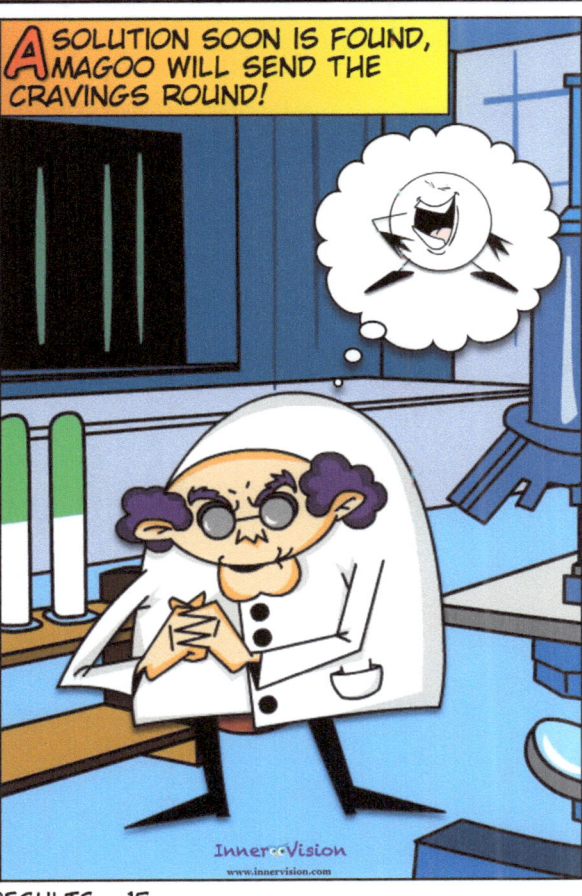

**A**SOLUTION SOON IS FOUND, MAGOO WILL SEND THE CRAVINGS ROUND!

Inner Vision
www.innervision.com

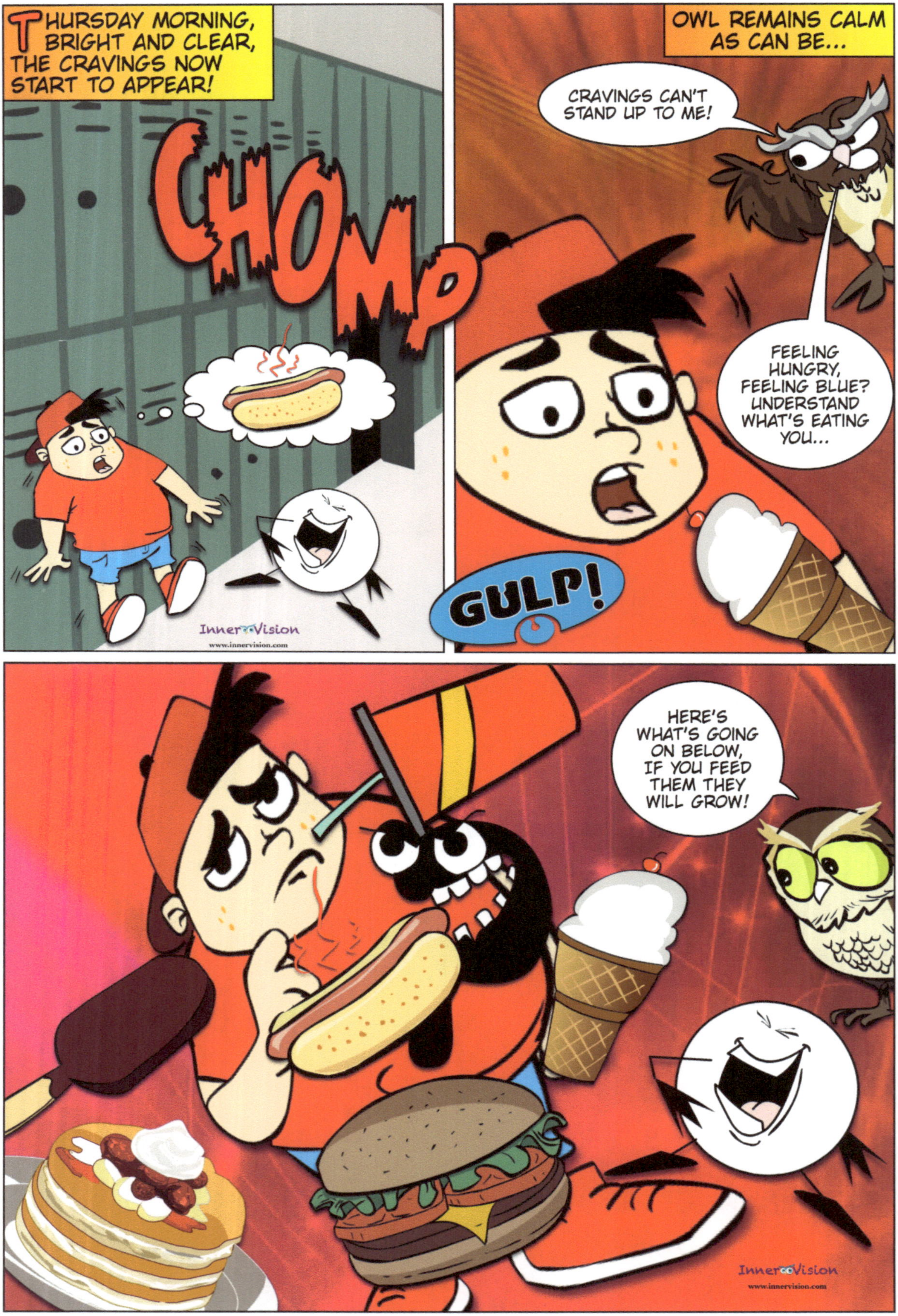
THURSDAY MORNING, BRIGHT AND CLEAR, THE CRAVINGS NOW START TO APPEAR!
CHOMP
InnerVision
www.innervision.com
OWL REMAINS CALM AS CAN BE...
CRAVINGS CAN'T STAND UP TO ME!
FEELING HUNGRY, FEELING BLUE? UNDERSTAND WHAT'S EATING YOU...
GULP!
HERE'S WHAT'S GOING ON BELOW, IF YOU FEED THEM THEY WILL GROW!
InnerVision
www.innervision.com

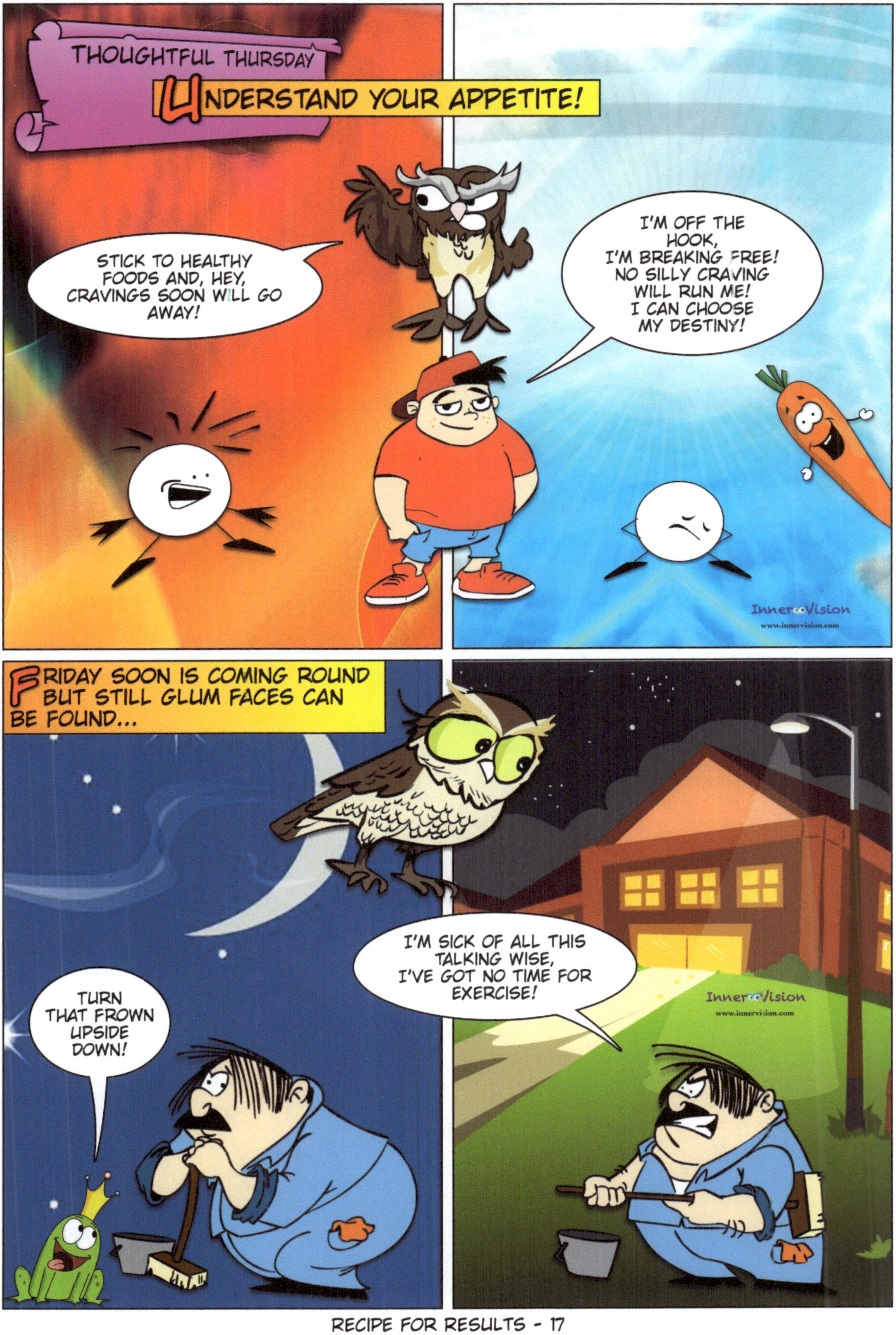
THOUGHTFUL THURSDAY
UNDERSTAND YOUR APPETITE!
STICK TO HEALTHY FOODS AND, HEY, CRAVINGS SOON WILL GO AWAY!
I'M OFF THE HOOK, I'M BREAKING FREE! NO SILLY CRAVING WILL RUN ME! I CAN CHOOSE MY DESTINY!
InnerVision
www.innervision.com
FRIDAY SOON IS COMING ROUND BUT STILL GLUM FACES CAN BE FOUND...
TURN THAT FROWN UPSIDE DOWN!
I'M SICK OF ALL THIS TALKING WISE, I'VE GOT NO TIME FOR EXERCISE!
InnerVision
www.innervision.com

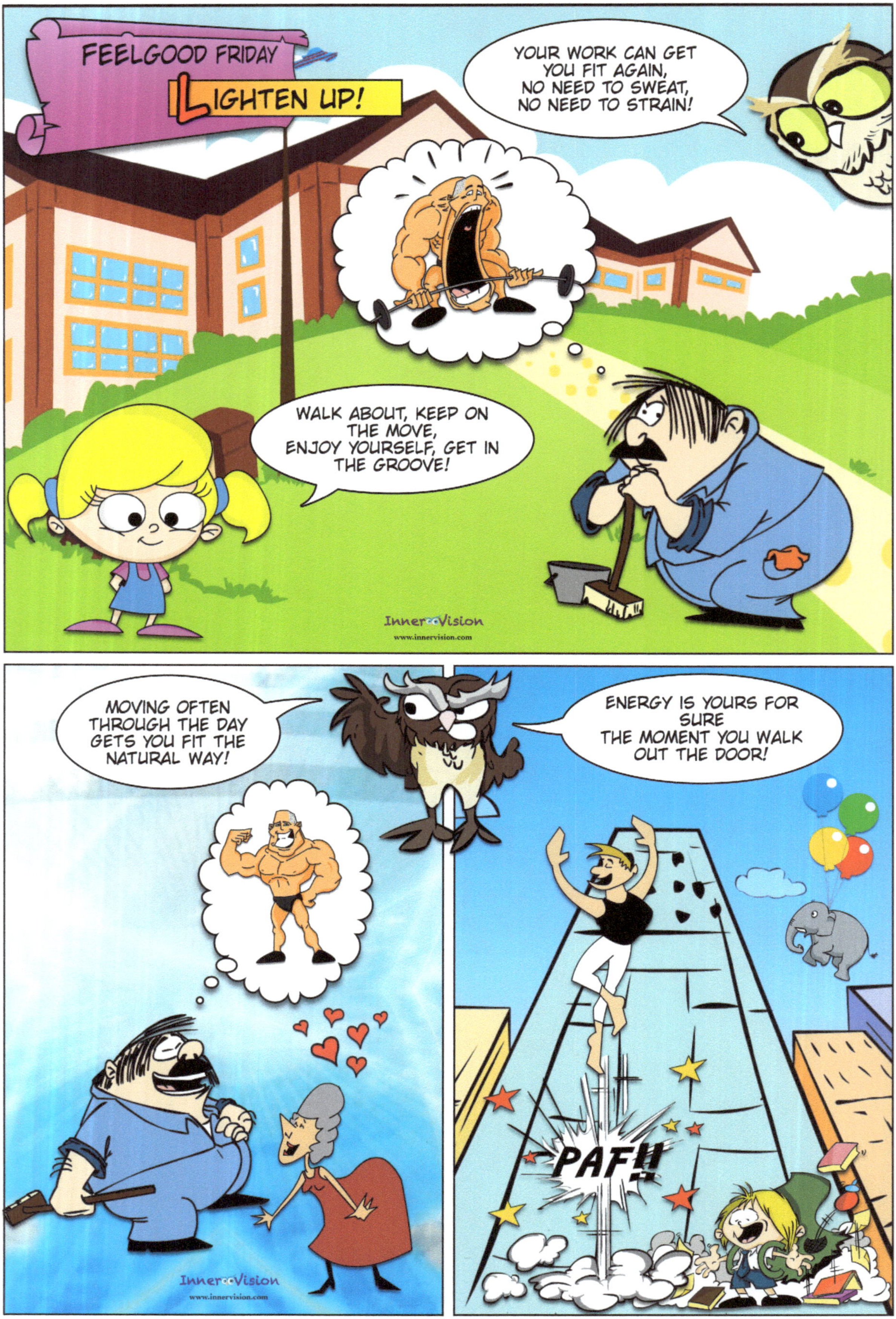

FEELGOOD FRIDAY
**LIGHTEN UP!**

YOUR WORK CAN GET YOU FIT AGAIN, NO NEED TO SWEAT, NO NEED TO STRAIN!

WALK ABOUT, KEEP ON THE MOVE, ENJOY YOURSELF, GET IN THE GROOVE!

MOVING OFTEN THROUGH THE DAY GETS YOU FIT THE NATURAL WAY!

ENERGY IS YOURS FOR SURE THE MOMENT YOU WALK OUT THE DOOR!

*PAF!!*

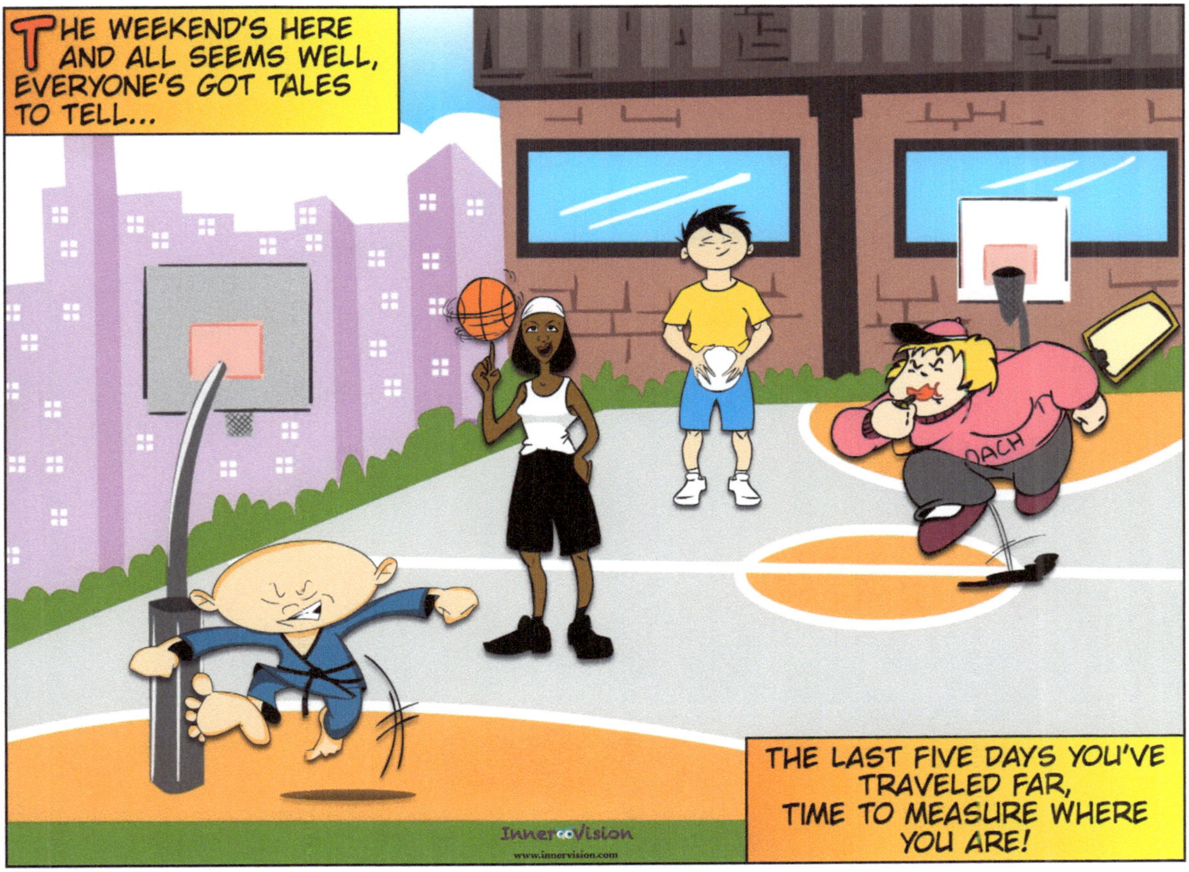

THE WEEKEND'S HERE AND ALL SEEMS WELL, EVERYONE'S GOT TALES TO TELL...

THE LAST FIVE DAYS YOU'VE TRAVELED FAR, TIME TO MEASURE WHERE YOU ARE!

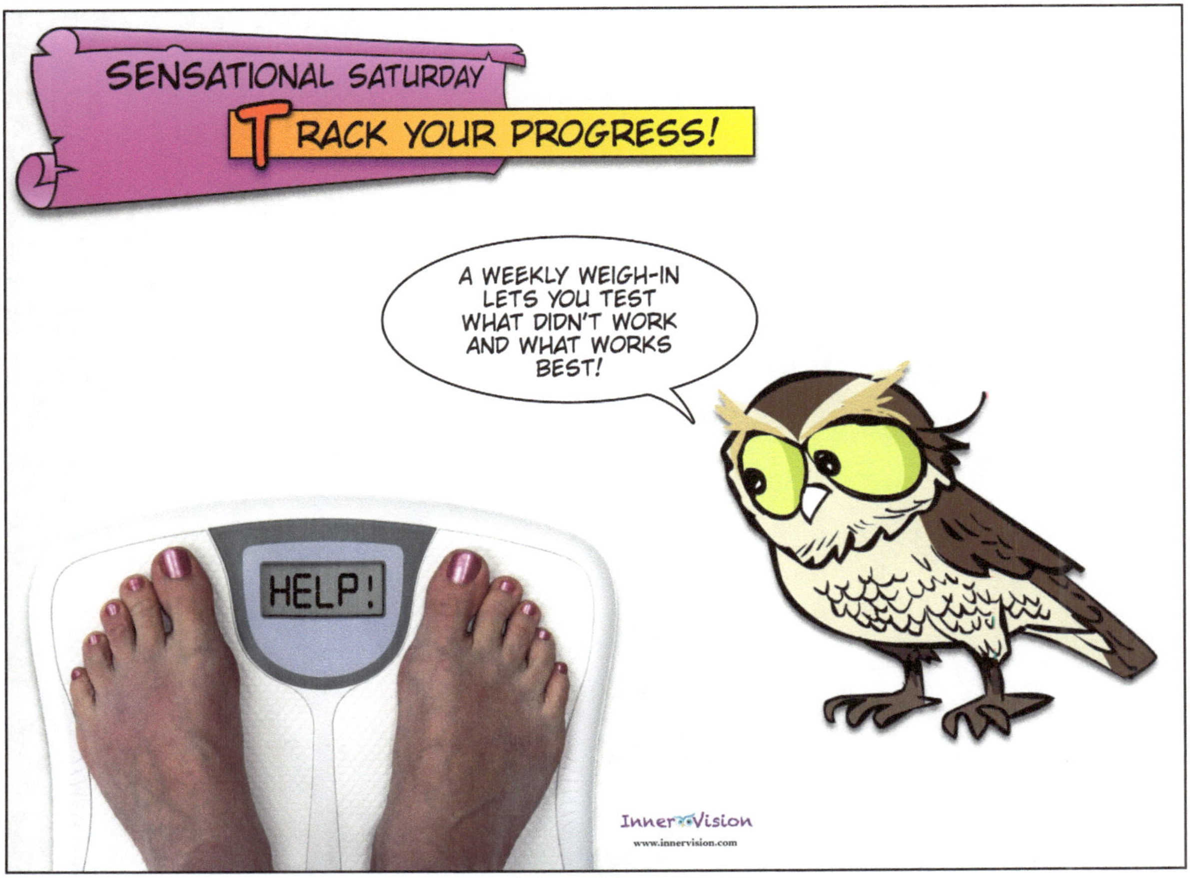

SENSATIONAL SATURDAY

TRACK YOUR PROGRESS!

A WEEKLY WEIGH-IN LETS YOU TEST WHAT DIDN'T WORK AND WHAT WORKS BEST!

HELP!

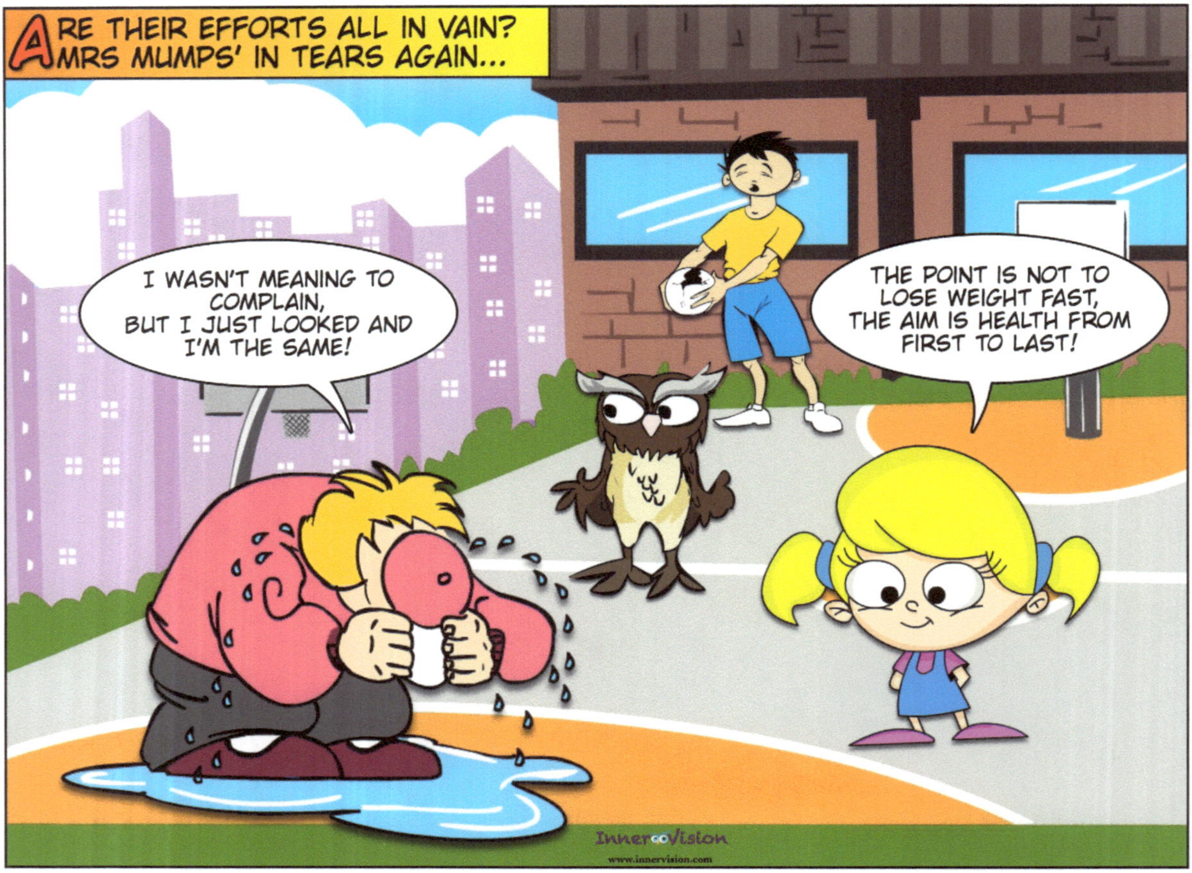
ARE THEIR EFFORTS ALL IN VAIN?
MRS MUMPS' IN TEARS AGAIN...
I WASN'T MEANING TO COMPLAIN, BUT I JUST LOOKED AND I'M THE SAME!
THE POINT IS NOT TO LOSE WEIGHT FAST, THE AIM IS HEALTH FROM FIRST TO LAST!
InnerVision
www.innervision.com

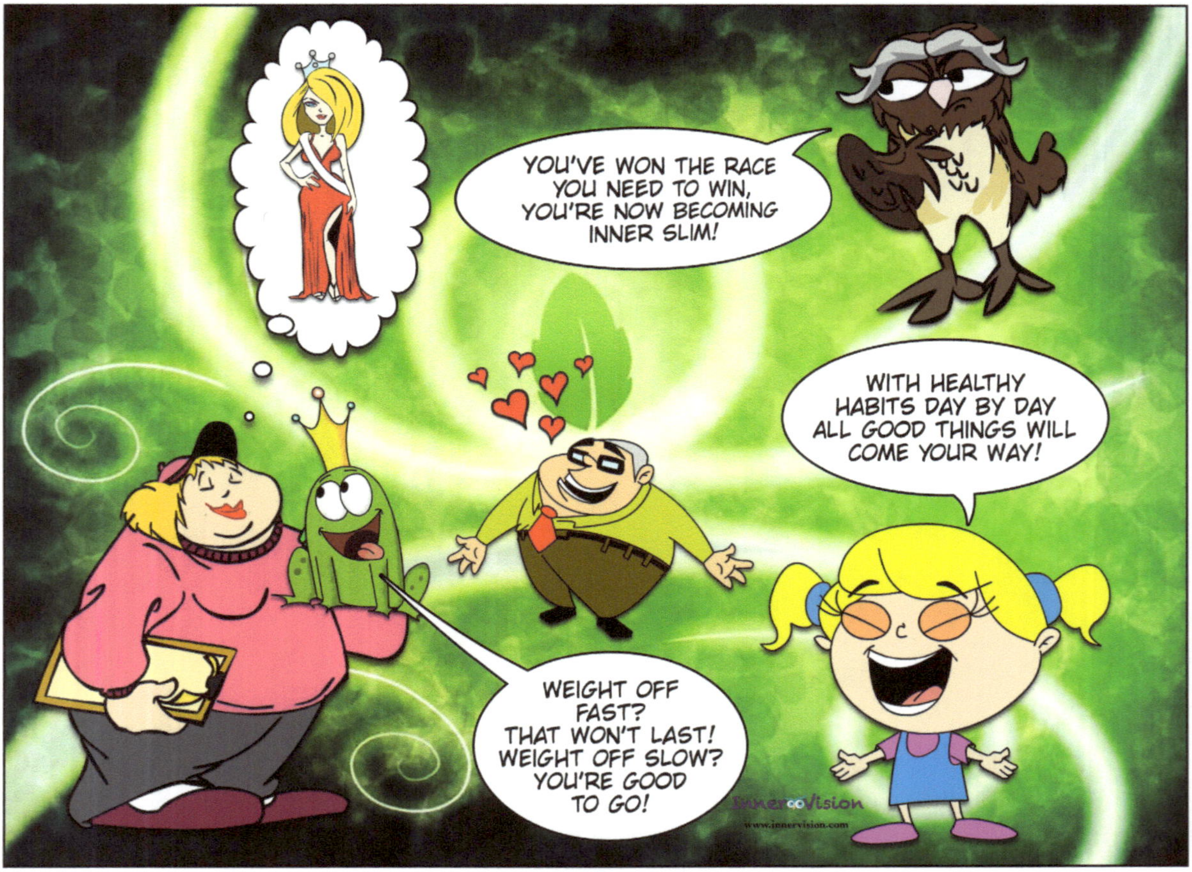
YOU'VE WON THE RACE YOU NEED TO WIN, YOU'RE NOW BECOMING INNER SLIM!
WITH HEALTHY HABITS DAY BY DAY ALL GOOD THINGS WILL COME YOUR WAY!
WEIGHT OFF FAST? THAT WON'T LAST! WEIGHT OFF SLOW? YOU'RE GOOD TO GO!
InnerVision
www.innervision.com

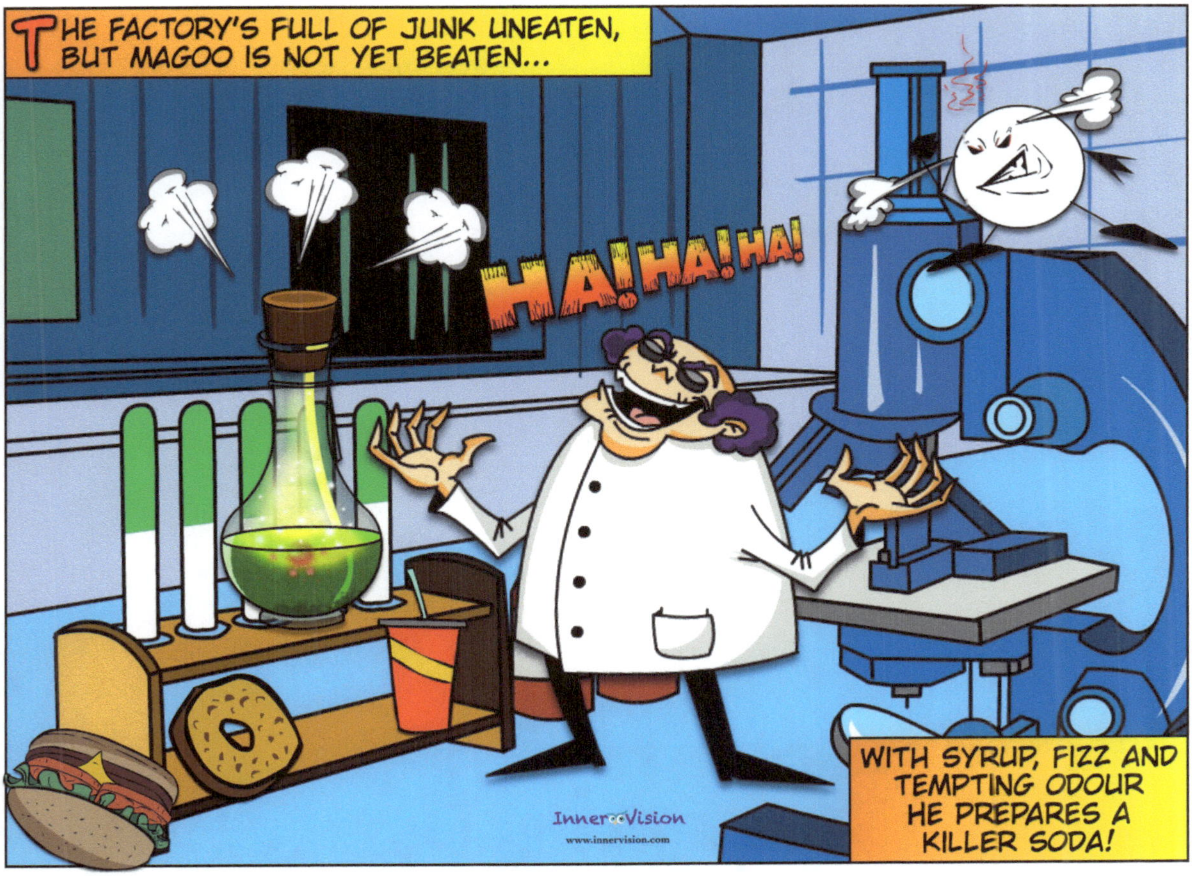

THE FACTORY'S FULL OF JUNK UNEATEN, BUT MAGOO IS NOT YET BEATEN...

HA! HA! HA!

WITH SYRUP, FIZZ AND TEMPTING ODOUR HE PREPARES A KILLER SODA!

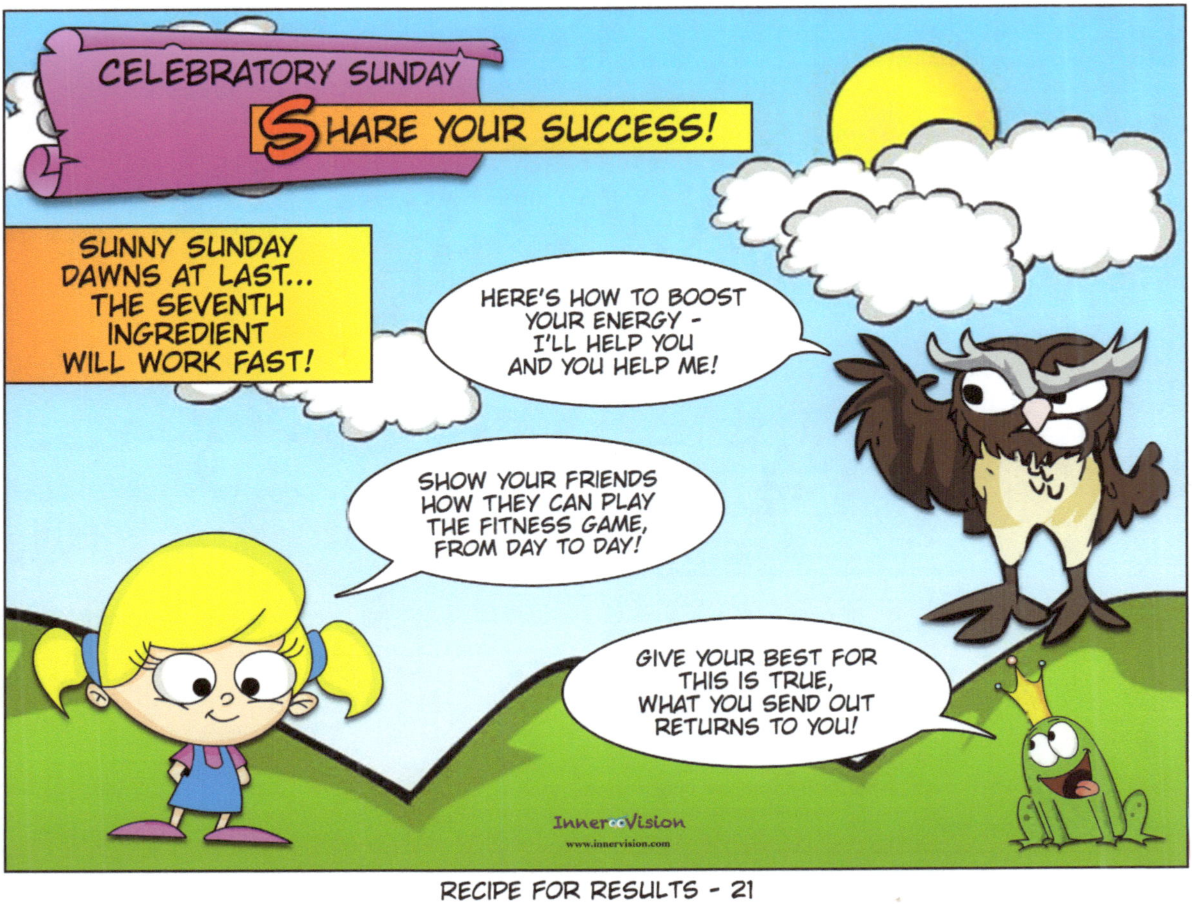

CELEBRATORY SUNDAY

SHARE YOUR SUCCESS!

SUNNY SUNDAY DAWNS AT LAST... THE SEVENTH INGREDIENT WILL WORK FAST!

HERE'S HOW TO BOOST YOUR ENERGY – I'LL HELP YOU AND YOU HELP ME!

SHOW YOUR FRIENDS HOW THEY CAN PLAY THE FITNESS GAME, FROM DAY TO DAY!

GIVE YOUR BEST FOR THIS IS TRUE, WHAT YOU SEND OUT RETURNS TO YOU!

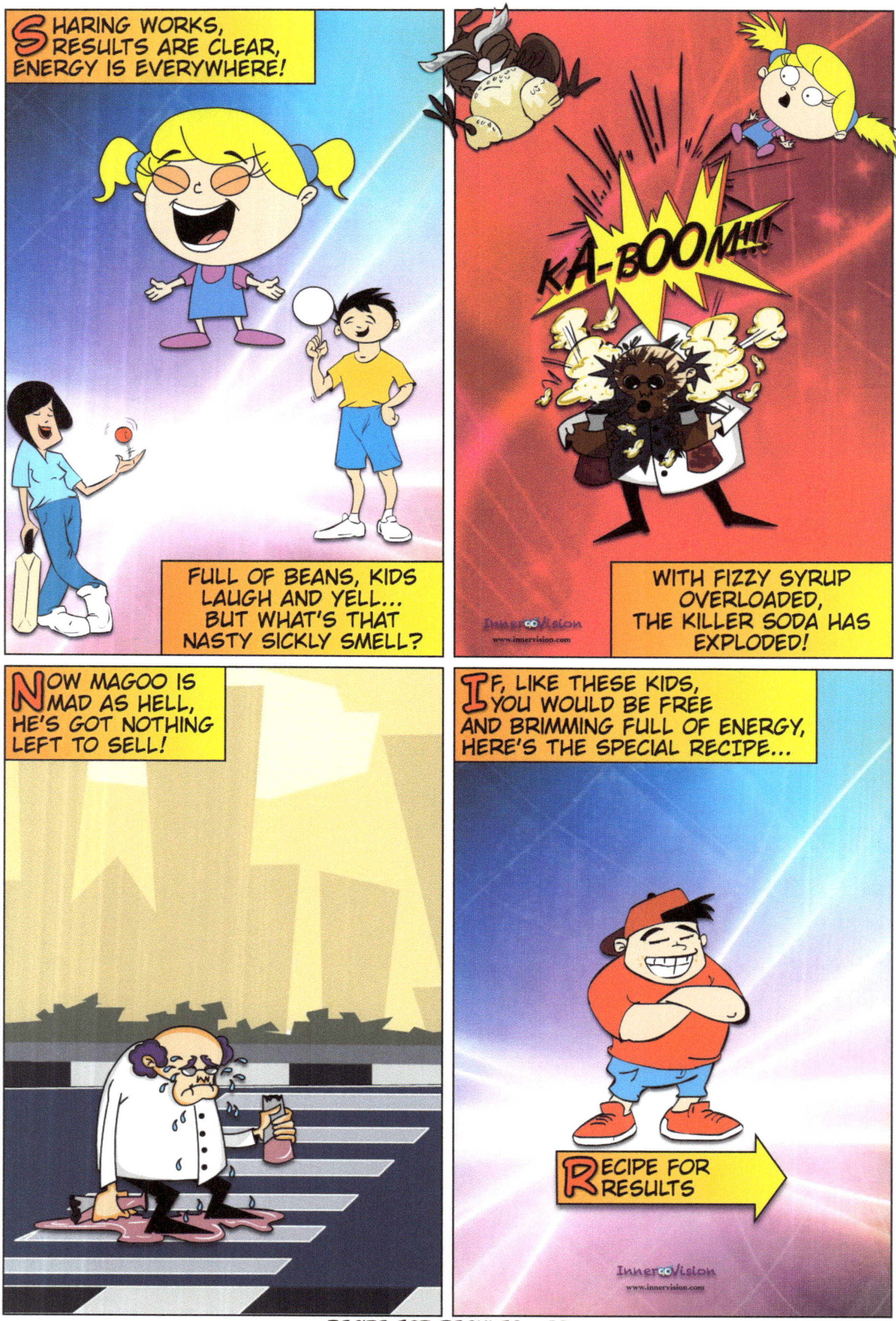

**SHARING WORKS, RESULTS ARE CLEAR, ENERGY IS EVERYWHERE!**

**FULL OF BEANS, KIDS LAUGH AND YELL... BUT WHAT'S THAT NASTY SICKLY SMELL?**

**KA-BOOM!!!**

**WITH FIZZY SYRUP OVERLOADED, THE KILLER SODA HAS EXPLODED!**

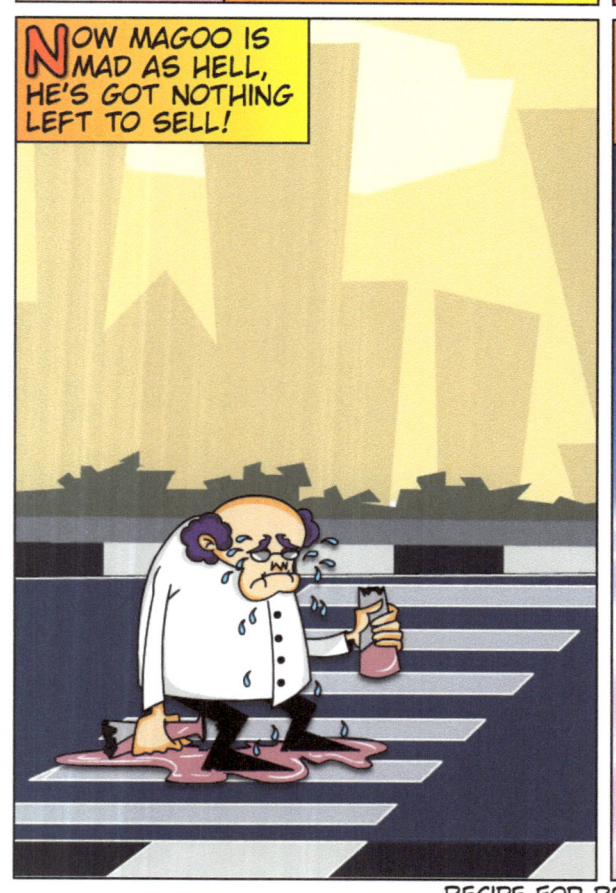

**NOW MAGOO IS MAD AS HELL, HE'S GOT NOTHING LEFT TO SELL!**

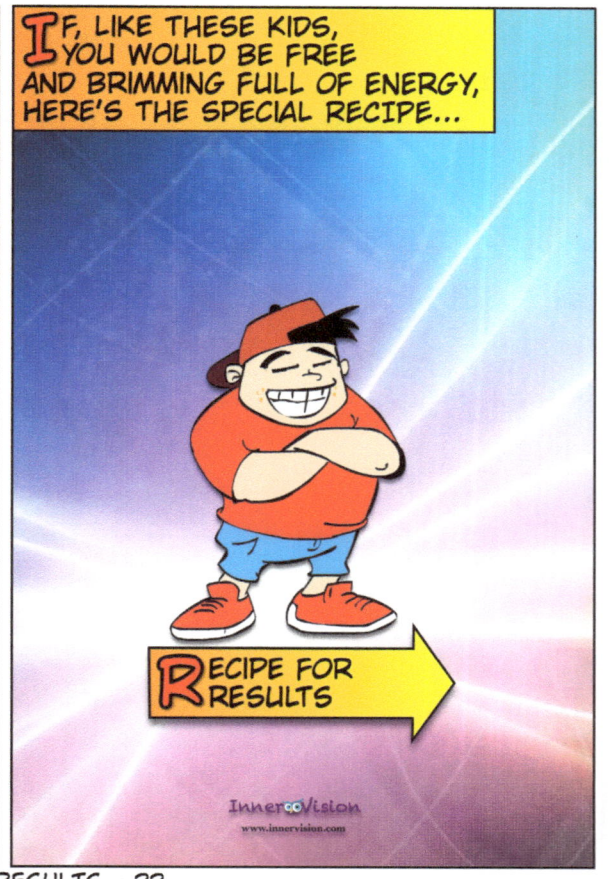

**IF, LIKE THESE KIDS, YOU WOULD BE FREE AND BRIMMING FULL OF ENERGY, HERE'S THE SPECIAL RECIPE...**

**RECIPE FOR RESULTS**

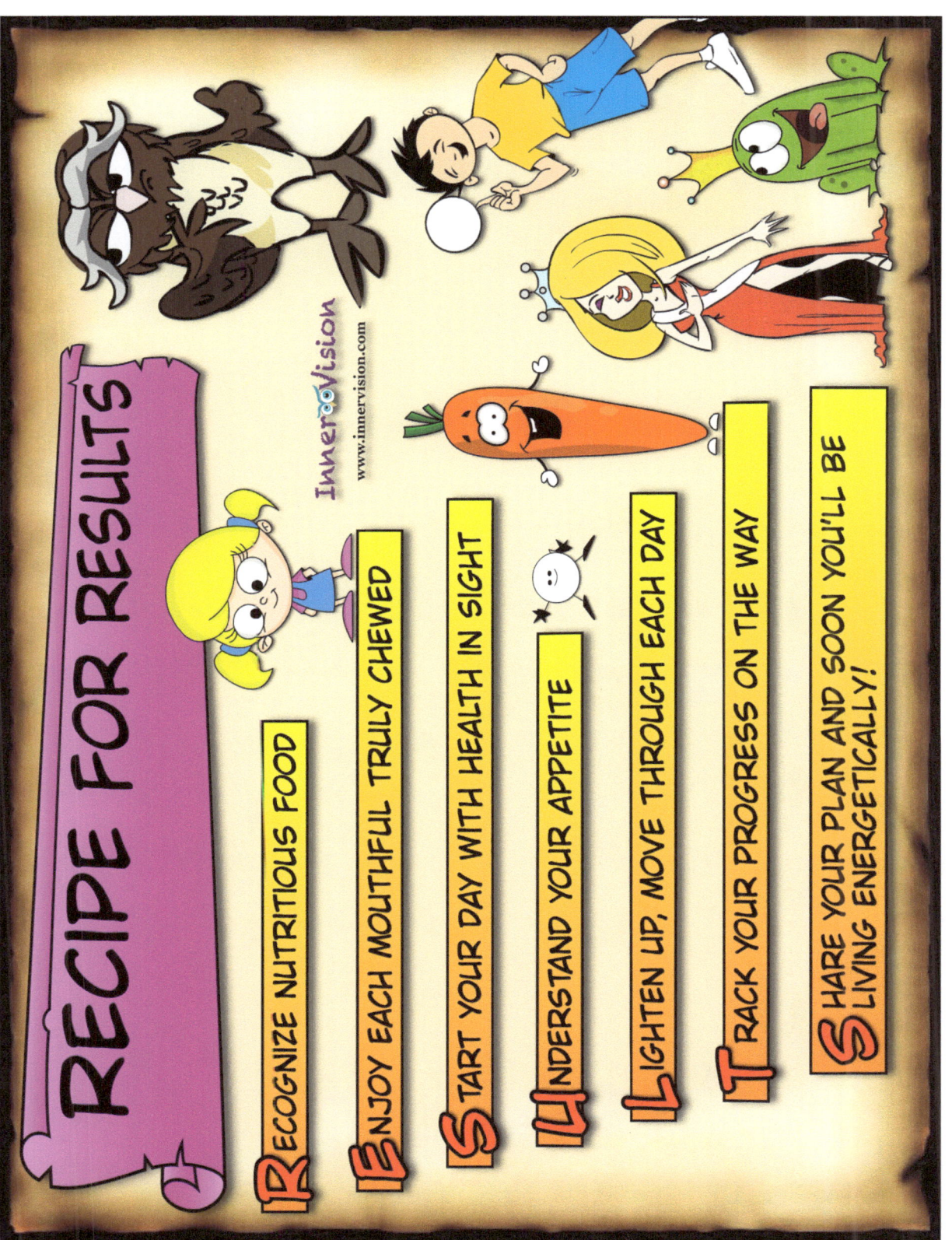

# RECIPE FOR RESULTS

**R**ECOGNIZE NUTRITIOUS FOOD

**E**NJOY EACH MOUTHFUL TRULY CHEWED

**S**TART YOUR DAY WITH HEALTH IN SIGHT

**U**NDERSTAND YOUR APPETITE

**L**IGHTEN UP, MOVE THROUGH EACH DAY

**T**RACK YOUR PROGRESS ON THE WAY

**S**HARE YOUR PLAN AND SOON YOU'LL BE LIVING ENERGETICALLY!

InnerVision
www.innervision.com

www.ingramcontent.com/pod-product-compliance
Lightning Source LLC
Chambersburg PA
CBHW060824290526
45792CB00005BB/1791